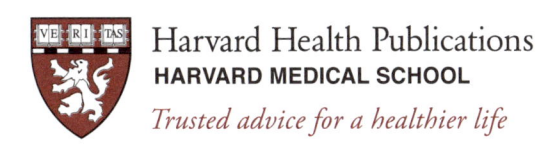

Harvard Health Publications
HARVARD MEDICAL SCHOOL
Trusted advice for a healthier life

Dear Reader,

Socrates may have said it best centuries ago when he noted, "To him whose feet hurt, everything hurts." It's hard to know whether the great philosopher suffered from worn-out joints, plantar fasciitis, bunions, or any number of painful foot ailments, but we do know two things: that he probably didn't wear supportive shoes—and that his words still ring true.

Foot problems can be structural (bunions, aching arches) or may result from a medical condition that affects the whole body (diabetes, obesity). You may not connect your foot woes to your waistline, but sometimes the two are related. Each time you take a step, about one and a half times your weight is placed on your foot. Every pound you gain in weight adds to the pounding on your feet. So don't be surprised if your foot care specialist asks how much you weigh the next time you develop a problem in one or both feet.

Foot problems develop for all sorts of reasons. All told, more than three out of four Americans will suffer some kind of foot ailment in their lifetimes. The most recent figures available from the American Academy of Orthopaedic Surgeons show that about 9.6 million people see a physician for foot pain or a foot injury each year. And there are more than 300 types of foot problems that can develop.

For the most part, foot problems are annoying, painful, and sometimes disabling, but they are rarely life-threatening. The most frequent foot problems include blisters, bunions, corns, and ingrown toenails. At times, however, untreated foot problems can have life-altering consequences, especially for the many Americans with diabetes. About 15% of people with diabetes will develop a foot ulcer, which, in some cases, can lead to complications that require amputating a toe or foot.

On the bright side, you can prevent and treat many foot problems by choosing comfortable, well-fitting shoes. Moreover, you can catch most foot problems early, when they are most effectively treated. If surgery does become necessary, surgical techniques have improved to the point where most foot operations are now done on an outpatient basis. In some cases, recovery times have become shorter. Still, recovery is often a prolonged process, typically from three to six months—and sometimes longer—to regain full functioning after most surgical procedures involving the foot.

This report will help you recognize and treat common foot ailments. It also discusses circumstances that require special care, including diabetes, vascular problems, and nerve disorders. Most important, it provides the information you need to walk comfortably and confidently for many years to come.

Sincerely,

Christopher P. Chiodo, M.D.
Medical Editor

James P. Ioli, D.P.M.
Medical Editor

Harvard Health Publications | Harvard Medical School | 10 Shattuck Street, Second Floor | Boston, MA 02115

The fantastic foot

Leonardo da Vinci once called the foot a "masterpiece of engineering and a work of art." Da Vinci's observation still holds true today under the harsher light of modern science: the human foot is an immensely practical, beautifully designed structure built to bear many times its weight thousands of times a day and bounce back ready for more.

One reason for the foot's amazing resilience is its ingenious design: it's meant to take a lot of pressure and wear and tear. Your foot has the sophisticated construction of a suspension bridge and the stability of a marble pedestal. Although it's one of the smaller parts of your body, the foot contains 28 different bones. Together, your two feet contain more than a quarter of all the bones in your body.

Foot structure

Your foot consists of three main components: the forefoot (the toes and ball of your foot), the midfoot (the arch), and the hindfoot (the heel). The underlying bone structure is intricate and complex (see Figure 1). For

Figure 1 A look at the foot

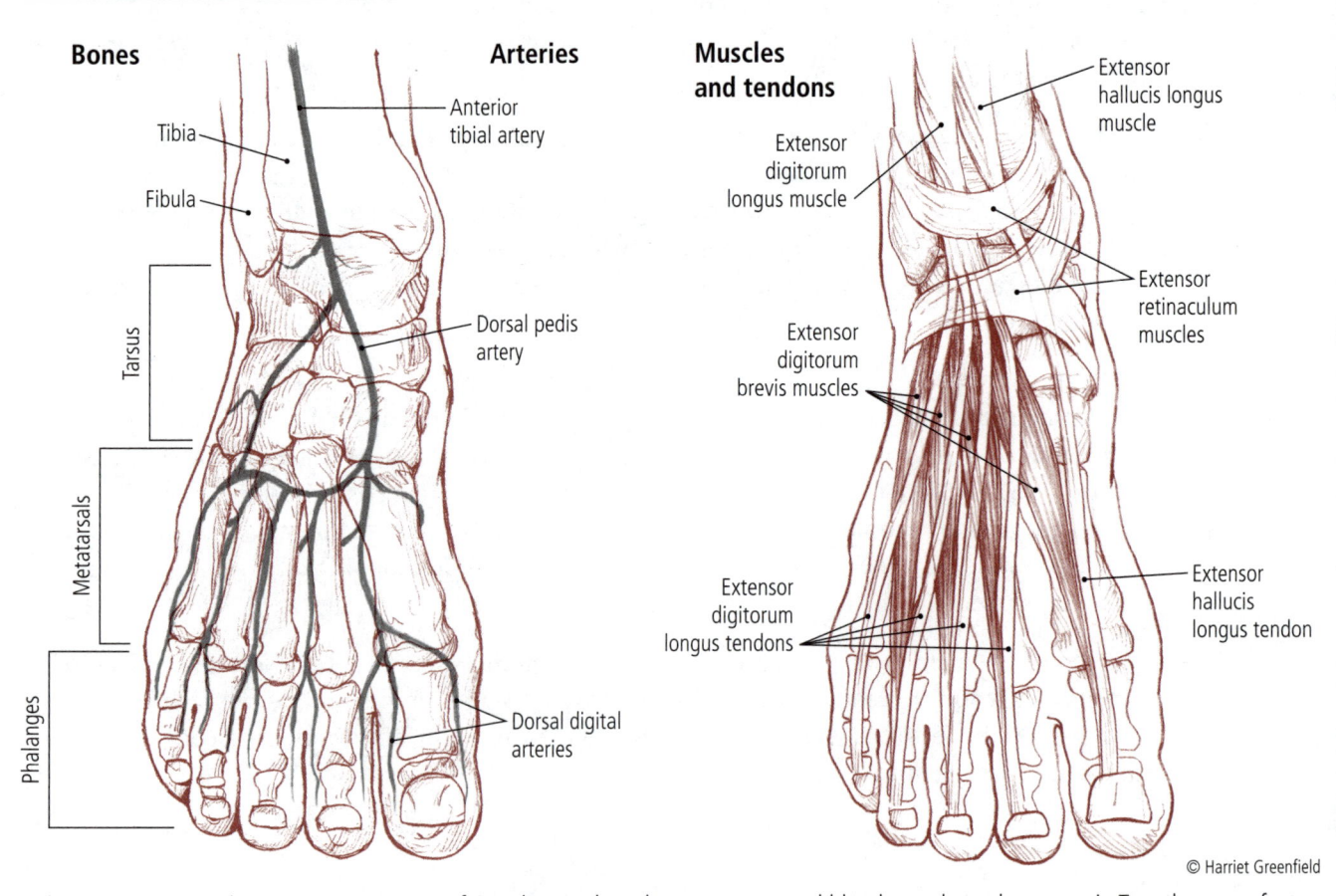

With every step you take, an intricate system of muscles, tendons, bones, nerves, and blood vessels works as a unit. Together, your feet contain 56 bones, 66 joints, and more than 200 tendons, muscles, and ligaments, as well as blood vessels and nerves. Because of this intricate structure, the human foot can sustain decades of use with remarkable resilience, especially with the support of roomy, well-cushioned shoes.

example, in each foot, your five toes contain 14 bones (two in your big toe and three each in the other four) called phalanges. Five longer bones, known collectively as the metatarsals, lead to the toes. Hidden under the base of the big toe are two tiny bones called sesamoids, which work like pulleys, enhancing the function of muscles and tendons and increasing the strength of the big toe.

The midfoot consists of five rectangular bones (three cuneiforms, the cuboid, and the navicular), which are short and broad and fit tightly together. Your hindfoot contains the largest bones in the foot, including the heel bone, or calcaneus, and the talus, located between the heel bone and the two bones of the lower leg.

In addition to its underlying bone structure, each foot has more than 100 muscles, tendons, and ligaments. The muscles move the bones, the tendons attach the muscles to the bones, and the ligaments connect the bones and help stabilize joints. Two soft-tissue structures are worth noting, since they have such vital functions. A ligament-like structure called the plantar fascia runs from your heel to the ball of your foot. It is one of the strongest connective tissues in the body, but it is prone to inflammation. The Achilles' tendon, which runs up the back of your foot, is the major connection between your foot and the muscles in your calf. This tendon enables you to lift your heel up so that your weight shifts to your toes—an essential function in walking and running. When injured, it can cause terrible pain and disability.

Your walking gait

Each step you take involves these components working together in precisely timed harmony. When you stand still, your weight is evenly distributed along your foot, and the plantar fascia is partially relaxed. As you walk, your heel touches the ground first,

▶ Finding help when problems develop

No matter how fantastic their design, feet often develop problems, especially as you age. Some foot problems can be managed by your primary care physician, who may prescribe medication or physical therapy, but often your doctor may diagnose the problem and refer you to one of several specialists, such as the following:

Podiatrist. A specialist in the medical, surgical, and orthopedic management of foot and ankle disorders. A podiatrist completes four years of podiatric medical school to earn a Doctor of Podiatric Medicine (D.P.M.) degree. Podiatrists go on to complete two to three years of hospital residency training, with an emphasis on foot and ankle surgery.

Orthopedist. A medical doctor (M.D.) who is also a surgeon specializing in musculoskeletal problems, including those of the bones, joints, tendons, and nerves of the foot and ankle. Orthopedists complete four years of medical school followed by several years of hospital residency in orthopedic surgery.

absorbing the impact of your weight. As the rest of your foot reaches the ground, your weight shifts forward to the ball of your foot and your toes. Meanwhile, your arch partially flattens and the plantar fascia is stretched. Then, your weight shifts again as you begin to rise on your toes and the ball of your foot—with the Achilles' tendon lifting your ankle—and your body is propelled over that foot, with the weight passing onto the other foot.

This gait cycle describes the mechanics of the way you walk. It starts when one heel strikes the ground and ends a few seconds later when that same heel hits the ground again. Foot care specialists often analyze a patient's gait cycle to look for structural and functional problems. For instance, if your arch flattens too much when you walk, your foot may be turning too far inward. This may be a sign of (or may cause) one of several foot disorders.

Your age in miles

When it comes to your feet, age is more about the number of miles you've logged than the number of birthdays you've celebrated. Although the foot undergoes certain changes associated with the natural process of aging, the amount of wear and tear it experiences depends more on your lifestyle and choice of shoes.

Imagine an automobile that you use to commute 50 miles daily, over busy roads full of potholes. That car will suffer more wear and tear than a similar car of the same age that you drive only occasionally and mostly on highways. The same is true of your feet. Some wear and tear comes from age, but much of it depends on mileage—that is, your activity level—and your footwear. Your weight, too, affects foot health. The more you weigh, the more wear and tear on your feet.

In other words, you can suffer foot pain and problems at any age. Even a 25-year-old can develop bunions, especially if there is a family history of the condition. Still, it helps to understand the normal changes that occur throughout life. Keep in mind that if you've been an avid athlete or have spent your adult life pushing your feet into high heels a half-size too small, your feet may be chronologically older than you are. Consider the following stages as guidelines, not hard-and-fast rules.

> ### Pain relief: Building foot strength
>
> Wearing supportive sneakers or shoes, stand with both feet flat. Lift off your heels onto your toes. Lower flat to the ground. Repeat 10 times. Pause. Perform five sets of 10 daily.
>
> After two weeks, if your feet are strong and uninjured, you can increase the intensity by performing the same set of exercises but standing on only one foot at a time. Rest the other foot gently on the back of your ankle. Hold the back of a chair or table for stability.

Birth to age 30

An infant or toddler's foot has an enviable amount of fat padding underneath it, partly to protect bones that are still forming. Indeed, the bones in a baby's foot are initially composed of cartilage, the same flexible substance that lines joints and is found in ears and noses. Some of the bones do not completely form until the late teens. As children grow and begin to walk, they develop an arch, and their feet strengthen. Feet are generally strong, supple, and problem-free through the third decade of life. This is why so many people in their 20s are able to dance the night away or run a 10-mile race without physical consequences or regrets.

30s and 40s

In your 30s and 40s, your feet undergo age-related changes like the rest of your body. Muscles weaken; tendons and ligaments become less resilient. You lose some of your natural shock absorption. Although your feet may start to bother you by your mid-30s, it's generally in the 40s that real problems develop. Typically, you may begin to notice that your feet ache at the end of the day, especially the heels, arches, and balls of your feet. For some people, this may be the time that bunions or hammertoes begin to emerge. This is also the time when nail fungus becomes more common. Your feet become more susceptible to injury as well as to aches and pains. If your feet are otherwise healthy, your best strategy is to exercise. The right exercises will stretch and strengthen your muscles and keep tendons and ligaments supple (see "Practice foot fitness," page 8).

Age 50 and over

By the time you reach your 50th birthday, you've probably also reached another milestone: you've put

75,000 miles on your feet. You may reach this milestone much earlier if you've led a foot-active lifestyle. By age 50, you may have lost nearly half of the fatty padding on the soles of your feet. You may also be wearing a shoe that's a size bigger than what you wore in your 20s, in part because of weight gain that puts greater pressure on your feet, and in part because your ligaments and tendons have lost some of their elasticity. If you are a mother, you have another reason for the increase in shoe size: hormones released during pregnancy also cause ligaments to relax.

Menopause can affect foot health. Unless countered by medications or exercise, the loss of estrogen and other hormonal changes can lower bone density, possibly leading to osteoporosis. This condition can raise the risk of stress fractures in any of the bones of the foot. Stress fractures are hairline breaks in the bone; unless treated appropriately, they can worsen and cause the bones to shift out of place.

As you move into your 50s, 60s, and beyond, it is important to take steps to offset problems that could become disabling. Studies evaluating older people who live in a community setting show that 20% to 30% of seniors have chronic foot pain. Causes include bunions, corns, and calluses, along with the onset of systemic problems such as diabetes, obesity, and osteoarthritis. Years of wearing shoes that don't fit properly is also a contributor. Foot problems in seniors increase the risk of falls and lead to pain in other areas of the body, flattened feet, limited range of motion in the ankle joint, and even depression. A 2010 study showed that among people over age 60, those who experienced a fall were more likely to have been bothered by foot pain.

It's wise to wear comfortable supportive shoes, over-the-counter cushioning shoe inserts, or both when you plan to increase your activity level (for example, in exercises such as walking, running, or tennis). It may also be time to consider alternative forms of exercise, such as swimming or bicycling, which put less pressure on the joints of the foot. Maintaining some form of exercise routine is vital to help offset problems later. At the same time, your skin may begin to dry out. Unless you moisturize your feet on a regular basis with creams or lotions, you may develop cracks and fissures in the skin. Not only is this painful, but it can also make you more susceptible to viruses and bacteria that enter through breaks in the skin and cause infection.

Caring for the older foot

Just like the rest of your body, your feet change with age. The skin grows thinner and drier; the nails may become thicker or more brittle. If nails are thick and yellow, it may indicate a health problem. Keep your feet healthy. Exercise or massage your feet to increase circulation. Pay attention to nutrition, too—maintaining overall good health, including eating well, helps your feet stay healthy along with the rest of you.

Another good idea is to moisturize feet regularly. Many people apply skin lotion to their bodies after a shower and forget their feet. Pay special attention to the heels, as these can get very dry. However, try not to apply lotion or cream in between your toes, as this area tends to be moist, and you may end up encouraging some type of fungal or bacterial growth. You can also apply moisturizer, cuticle oil, or vitamin E oil to your nails, which will help soften the cuticles—the thin layer of skin at the bottom and sides of your toenail—although there's no evidence that it will keep your nails healthy or make them grow faster. Or try a pedicure to pamper your feet.

If you wear nail polish regularly, you may notice that your toenails seem yellow when you remove the polish. This problem can also affect fingernails, but it seems more pronounced with toenails, perhaps because people tend to redo their toenails less frequently than their fingernails. To reduce yellowing, remove the nail polish once a week and let your nails "breathe" for a day or two before you polish them again.

Helpful hint

As people grow older, nails may become thicker, making them harder to cut. Here's a home remedy that works: apply a bit of Vicks VapoRub ointment (normally used for easing chest congestion) to your thick nails, massaging it on gently. Wipe off any excess ointment before pulling on socks or going to bed. After a month or so of daily applications, you should find your toenails softer and easier to trim. It's not clear why this works, but one of the ingredients in Vicks VapoRub (probably the eucalyptus oil) apparently softens the nails and makes them easier to cut.

SPECIAL SECTION

Keeping your feet healthy

Jammed in a hot shoe all day, taking the brunt of your daily travels, the foot is often overlooked when it comes to health and fitness. But once it starts to hurt, it will quickly remind you of your neglect. Women's feet, in particular, suffer from the stress and abuse of tight, high-heeled shoes, with the result that women are more likely than men to suffer from nearly all foot problems (see Figure 2). Foot fitness can help you avoid disability later in life, keeping you active and engaged.

Many of the same things you do to maintain your overall health can also help your feet stay healthy. But two lifestyle factors stand out as particularly foot-healthy: maintaining a healthy weight, and keeping your feet in good physical condition with stretching and exercise.

8 steps to foot health

Here are some basic steps to help prevent many foot problems:

1. Buy shoes that fit well, with low heels and plenty of room for your toes (see "What to look for in a shoe," page 45).
2. Maintain a healthy weight. Excess weight increases the load on your feet and the risk of developing foot problems (see "Maintain a healthy weight," above).
3. Keep your feet clean and dry (see "Caring for your feet," page 33).
4. Trim toenails straight across (see "Ingrown toenails," page 24).
5. Wear sandals or shower shoes in locker rooms or public swimming pools (see "Toenail fungus," page 27, and "Athlete's foot," page 29).
6. Exercise your feet regularly (see "Practice for foot fitness," page 8).
7. Protect the skin of your feet from the sun's harmful ultraviolet rays (see "Protect your feet," page 37).
8. Inspect the skin of your feet routinely for changes (see "Skin cancer," page 36, and "Diabetes," page 33).

Maintain a healthy weight

Your weight plays a major role in your risk for many health problems: cardiovascular disease, high blood pressure, high cholesterol, diabetes, several forms of cancer, arthritis, gallstones, adult-onset asthma, infertility, sleep apnea, and even snoring. So it should come as no surprise that excess weight can also contribute to certain foot problems, by adding pounds to the pounding your feet take every day, and increasing the risk for atherosclerosis, poor circulation, and diabetes.

First of all, excess weight can contribute to the misery of common structural problems such as heel pain and arthritis. Any foot ailment hurts more with more weight on it. Many foot care specialists today ask about your height and weight, as well as other aspects of your health, before suggesting a therapy. If you are overweight or obese, you are likely to leave the doctor's office not only with pain medication and instructions for stretching exercises, but also with some suggestions on how to lose weight.

What determines whether

you're overweight or obese isn't the bathroom scale, but rather a scientific calculation of weight in relation to height called the body mass index, or BMI. More than two-thirds of American adults are either overweight (with a BMI of 25 to 29) or obese (with a BMI of 30 or higher), according to the Centers for Disease Control and Prevention.

Your weight is determined partly by genetics; some people are born with a tendency to be overweight. But you can control your weight to a considerable degree by limiting how much you eat and getting regular physical activity.

Choose a weight-loss plan

Many diet plans are based on the premise that certain foods are better than others for helping you lose weight. But although certain foods are healthier than others, the key to losing weight is eating fewer calories than you burn each day. Weight-loss experts have learned that diet plans that emphasize certain foods or food combinations actually work by lowering your calorie consumption. No study has shown that any diet that restricts or advocates a particular type of food helps you lose weight without calorie reduction.

Very simply, to lose weight, you have to limit total calories and be active enough to burn those calories on a daily, ongoing basis. So choose a diet plan that you can stick with, and calorie reduction will likely result. Harvard nutrition researchers do not endorse any single diet plan, but they do recommend a three-pronged strategy for losing weight, as follows.

Be physically active. Aim for at least 30 minutes of strenuous physical activity (such as fast swimming) or an hour of moderate activity (such as walking briskly) on most days—more if you want to lose weight faster. But protect your feet with well-cushioned, supportive shoes. Exercise not only burns calories, but it also builds muscle, or at least prevents muscle loss. This is important because the more muscle you have in relation to fat tissue, the higher your resting metabolism—the rate at which your body burns energy when you're at rest. And the higher your resting metabolism, the more calories you burn. Exercise also helps prevent insulin resistance, a cause of diabetes and high cholesterol.

Figure 2 Types of foot pain in men and women

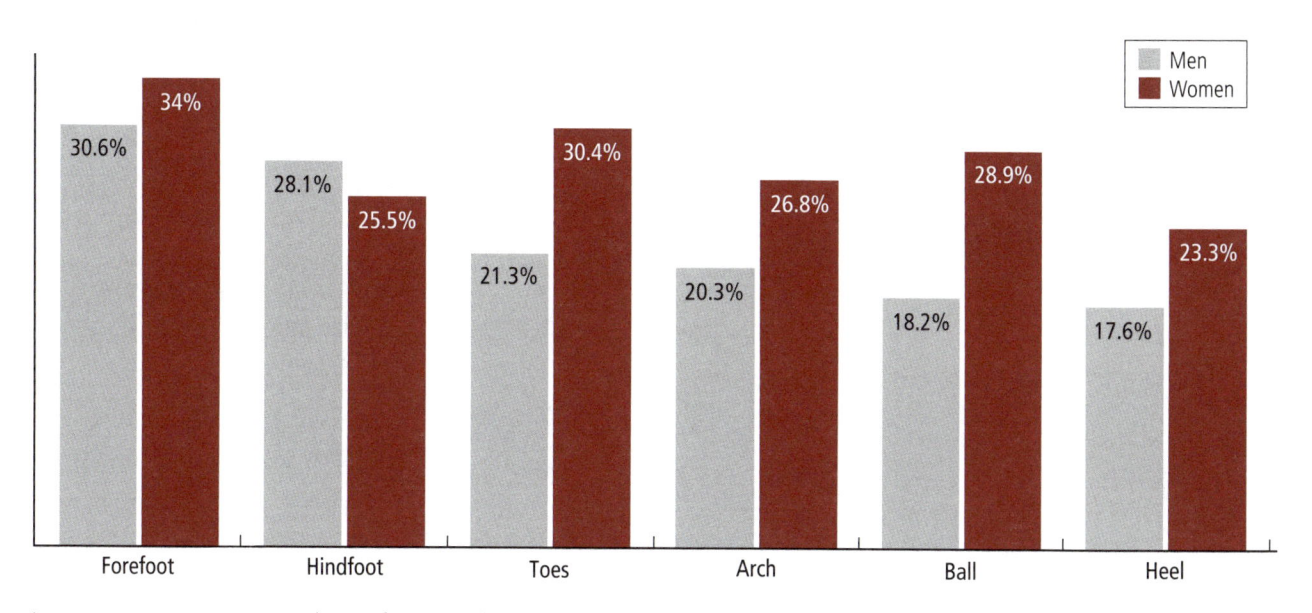

Category	Men	Women
Forefoot	30.6%	34%
Hindfoot	28.1%	25.5%
Toes	21.3%	30.4%
Arch	20.3%	26.8%
Ball	18.2%	28.9%
Heel	17.6%	23.3%

In one survey, women reported more foot pain than men in all but one category. *Adapted from C.L. Hill,* Journal of Foot and Ankle Research, *2008.*

SPECIAL SECTION | Keeping your feet healthy

Find a diet that works for you. No single diet plan works for everyone, but if you follow a few general guidelines, you'll be well on your way to eating better so that you can meet your nutritional needs even as you try to cut calories. Nutrition experts at the Harvard School of Public Health emphasize that healthy eating means limiting your intake of white carbohydrates (such as white bread) and added sugars (soft drinks, candy, cookies). Instead, choose whole grains and plenty of fruits and vegetables. Eat relatively little meat, especially processed meats. Use olive oil and other vegetable oils instead of butter, margarine, hydrogenated oils, and other sources of saturated and trans fats.

Be a defensive eater. Learn to stop eating before you feel stuffed. In restaurants, avoid oversized portions, share an entrée, or choose an appetizer and salad instead of an entrée. Share or skip dessert, too. Look for hidden calories: an 8-ounce glass of cola has 100 calories. So does the same amount of grapefruit juice (although it's healthier because it has more nutrients). Better to drink mainly water or seltzer, which have no calories.

Practice foot fitness

Exercising your feet on a regular basis not only improves overall foot health, but may also reduce your risk for injury. Walking is the best overall foot exercise. When you walk, you put your foot through its full range of motion, from the time your heel hits the ground until you lift off with your toes. Moreover, walking is one of the best forms of exercise for your entire body. It improves your cardiovascular

---

Limber up
To limber up your foot before attempting other exercises, try this:

1. Sit in a chair with your feet flat on the floor.
2. Lift your left leg so your foot is off the floor and use your big toe to make circles in the air, moving in a clockwise direction, for 15 to 20 rotations.
3. Reverse direction and make another 15 to 20 circles, this time in a counter-clockwise direction.
4. Repeat with your right foot.

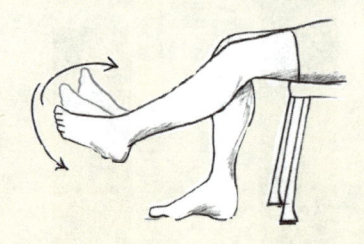

Bottom of foot
To stretch the muscles on the bottom of your feet:

1. Stand with feet together.
2. Step back with your left leg so your heel is raised and your toes press against the ground. You should feel the muscles on the bottom of your feet pull gently.
3. Hold for 20 to 30 seconds.
4. Repeat with your right foot.

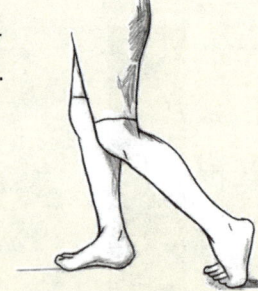

Top of foot
To stretch the muscles on top of your feet:

1. Stand on a phone book, which should be placed on a non-slippery floor (like a carpet), with the balls of your feet near the edge so your toes extend into free space.
2. Curl your toes slowly downward, as if you were trying to open the book. Hold for 20 to 30 seconds (or however long you can; you may need to build up to this). You should feel a pull on the top of your feet and toes.
3. Step off the book. Now, working with one foot at a time, raise your heel and curl your toes under, pressing the tops of your toes against the floor. You should feel the muscles on the top of your feet and the front of your ankle gently stretch.
4. Hold for 20 to 30 seconds.
5. Repeat with the other foot.

---

8 Foot Care Basics www.health.harvard.edu

Keeping your feet healthy | SPECIAL SECTION

health and can help your circulation, muscle tone, and mood.

Before walking, or doing any other exercise, take some time to stretch and strengthen the muscles in your feet. Otherwise, your feet will suddenly bear the brunt of all that activity, especially with high-impact sports like tennis or aerobics. If you're going to walk, be sure to stretch your legs and upper body in addition to your feet. Then hit the road—starting out slowly if it's the first time you've exercised in a while. Aim for 20 minutes three times a week, walking at a comfortable pace. If that's too strenuous, try walking for 10 to 15 minutes. Gradually, pick up the pace so that after five to 10 minutes you can still talk but are breathing more heavily than usual. At this point, you are achieving aerobic benefits.

Here are some other hints to make your walk more pleasant and to protect your feet:

- Make sure your shoes provide enough support but allow your feet to "breathe" (see "What to look for in a shoe," page 45).
- Walk with your head up and your back straight.
- You may swing your arms freely. If your fingertips tend to swell after a while, bend your arms at the elbow and swing your elbows gently at waist level, keeping your shoulders and arms relaxed.
- Start on level ground; work up to hills later.
- After walking, take time to cool down. You can do so with stretching exercises or, if you've been walking briskly, by walking at a slower pace.

If the shoe fits

If you're not wearing the proper

Achilles' tendon (runner's stretch)

To stretch your Achilles' tendon:

1. Stand at arm's length from a wall, pressing your hands against it and keeping your feet together.
2. Step back with your left leg, bending your right knee slightly and keeping the left heel on the ground. You should feel a stretch along your calf to your ankle. Hold for 20 to 30 seconds.
3. Repeat with your right leg.

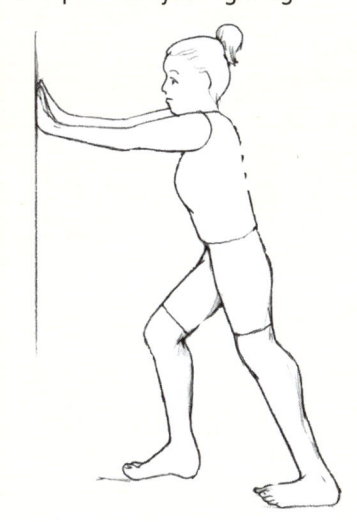

Ankle strength

You can practice a simple exercise to increase ankle strength that mimics the movement of your foot when you press down on an accelerator or clutch in a car:

1. Sit in a chair with your feet flat on the floor, pointing forward.
2. Lift your left leg. Hold the ends of an exercise band and place the center of the band under the ball of your foot.
3. Slowly press against the exercise band, as if you were stepping on the gas pedal of your car, and hold for a few seconds. You should feel a stretch on the upper part of your foot. Then release.
4. Repeat 10 to 15 times.
5. Repeat with your right leg.

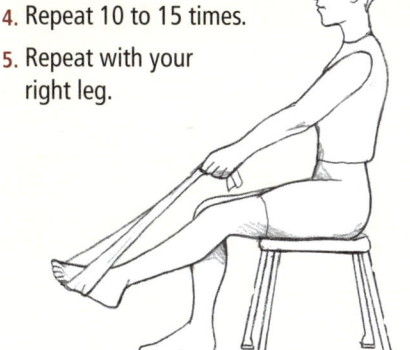

Heel exercises

To stretch the back of your heel:

1. Loop an exercise band around the leg of a heavy piece of furniture, such as a table or desk.
2. Sitting directly in front of it, slip your foot into the loop so the exercise band curls around your forefoot, just below your toes.
3. Pull back with your forefoot, flexing at the ankle. Hold for several seconds, then relax. You should feel a stretch along the back of your heel.
4. Repeat 10 to 15 times.
5. Repeat with your other foot.

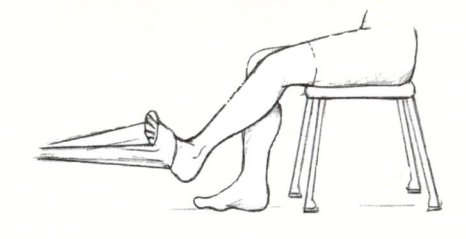

www.health.harvard.edu

Foot Care Basics

SPECIAL SECTION | Keeping your feet healthy

shoes while doing any strenuous exercise, you're leaving your feet vulnerable to injury. Choose sturdy, properly fitting athletic shoes that are roomy enough to support the width of your foot. Sports-specific athletic shoes are recommended if you are frequently involved in a single sport. Your shoes should hold your feet in the position that is most natural to the movement required for the sport. For instance, a running shoe is built to accommodate impact and the sole is designed for forward movement, so you wouldn't want to wear them to a tennis match, where you'll need to move side to side. That's a recipe for an ankle roll. A cross-training shoe may be a wise choice for someone who exercises moderately and participates in a variety of activities. Be sure to pay attention to your sneaker's shelf life. A worn-out shoe won't offer the protection you need.

Even when you are not exercising, wearing properly fitted, supportive shoes goes a long way toward keeping your feet healthy. For everyday wear, choose sturdy shoes that have adequate cushioning, a wide toe box, and flexibility at the ball of the foot. For detailed advice, see "Shoes for healthy feet," page 44.

Exercises for foot fitness

The exercises described in this section should take no longer than 15 to 20 minutes. It's best to start slowly. Once you get used to exercising, build it into a daily routine. You can even do these exercises during the workday. You can do some while you sit at your desk; others require you to stand up. To avoid slips and falls, you may want to do these exercises barefoot and have a chair, desk, or wall nearby that you can use for balance.

Don't do these exercises if they hurt. And if you have arthritis, diabetes, cardiovascular problems, or structural foot problems that might affect your ability to exercise, consult a foot care specialist first (see "Other health conditions," page 33).

Flexibility exercises. Exercises that improve flexibility help keep your feet limber and may reduce your risk for injury. Don't worry if your feet have grown stiff with age; studies show that no matter how old you are, you can still improve your flexibility. The easiest way to build flexibility is through slow and gentle daily stretches, focusing on one group of muscles at a time.

Resistance exercises. Resistance exercises are those in which your muscles work against some type of resistance, such as weights or exercise bands. Resistance exercises strengthen muscles, which, in turn, provide better support and protection for the foot as a whole. Exercise bands look a bit like compression bandages but come in various colors that correspond to the amount of resistance they provide.

Heels that hurt

Heel pain can take several forms (see Figure 3), but it usually develops when people overdo high-impact exercise or wear poorly fitting shoes. Some heel pain can be prevented by wearing supportive shoes with cushioned heels, by warming up before you exercise, and by avoiding excess weight gain as you grow older (see "Maintain a healthy weight," page 6). Here are a few of the most common sources of heel pain.

Plantar fasciitis and heel spurs

Inflammation of the plantar fascia—the ligament-like structure that runs from your heel to the ball of your foot—is a leading cause of heel pain, affecting two million people in the United States and accounting for one million doctor's visits annually. And it's no wonder; when too much pressure or strain is placed on the plantar fascia, it can become inflamed, usually at the heel. If you develop plantar fasciitis, you usually feel pain under your heel when you first get out of bed. The pain may ease as you walk around, only to return later in the day.

Heel spurs are abnormal growths of bone or calcium that can resemble a cowboy's spurs. They sometimes form on the back or bottom of the heel bone. Though their exact causes are unclear, some physicians believe that heel spurs develop when the plantar fascia pulls away from the heel from overuse or poor support, because you've gained weight, or because your arches have flattened. The heel spurs themselves don't cause pain, but sometimes they cause the plantar fascia or other tissues around the spur to degenerate and become inflamed and start to hurt.

▶ SYMPTOMS OF **Plantar fasciitis**

- Sharp pain with first steps in the morning, which eases after a few minutes
- Pain that returns in the afternoon or evening

Treating plantar fasciitis and heel spurs

Plantar fasciitis usually goes away on its own, but it may take awhile—anywhere from six weeks to a cumbersome 12 months. So treatments are typically aimed at speeding up relief, rather than correcting an anatomical problem. Although a wide range of treatment methods are available, a program of exercises specifically designed to stretch the plantar fascia has shown some success compared with other strategies (see "Plantar fascia–specific stretching exercise," page 12).

When pain first occurs, the best strategy is to rest a few days, gently stretch the foot, and apply ice. An over-the-counter or prescription pain reliever may also be helpful. Many pain relievers are nonsteroidal anti-inflammatory drugs (NSAIDs), which reduce swelling as well as pain (see Table 2, page 41). The immediate

Figure 3 Sites where structural problems occur

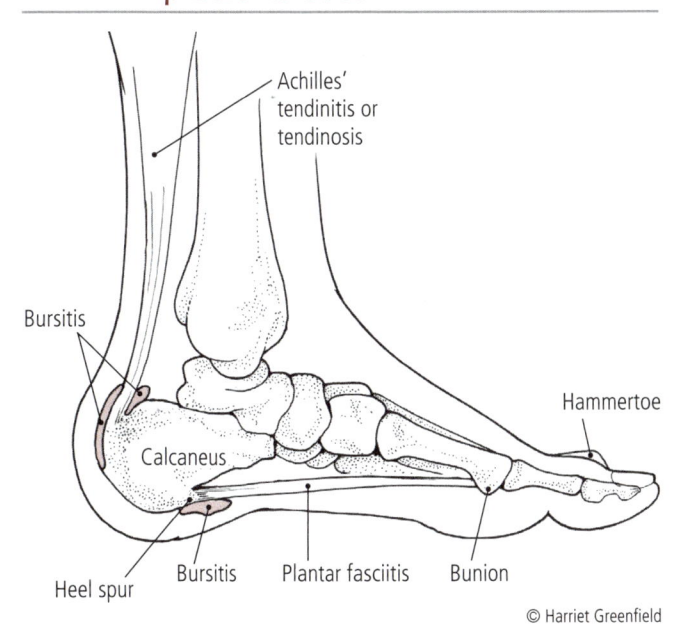

© Harriet Greenfield

The foot is a complex structure and can experience a variety of structural problems or injuries. Among the more common of these are Achilles' tendinitis, Achilles' tendinosis, bursitis, plantar fasciitis and heel spurs, bunions and bunionettes, and hammertoes.

pain should go away quickly, but it may take longer for the NSAIDs to reduce the inflammation. NSAID medications have a variety of side effects, so it is important to discuss your personal health risks with your doctor when considering long-term use of any of them.

You can also try purchasing over-the-counter cushion inserts and wearing supportive low-heeled (but not flat) shoes to ease the pressure on your heels. If you continue to experience discomfort after six to eight weeks, consult a foot care specialist, who may recommend stretching exercises, physical therapy, night splints, or a steroid injection to reduce pain and inflammation. Studies have shown no benefit to using custom orthotics for treating plantar fasciitis.

In extreme cases, surgery may be necessary, but this is recommended only if you are still experiencing substantial pain after six to 12 months and all other methods are exhausted. If so, the surgeon will remove the degenerated part of the plantar fascia to eliminate the pain. If a particularly large heel spur is present, it may be removed, but this is extremely rare. Endoscopy, a minimally invasive technique, can sometimes be used to release the plantar fascia. Potential complications from either an open or endoscopic procedure can include arch collapse or damage to a branch of the posterior tibial nerve, which can lead to persistent recurring pain. If you are considering surgery, you should discuss these risks with your doctor.

Some foot care specialists have begun using extracorporeal shock wave therapy to treat plantar fasciitis. Shock wave treatment entails one to three sessions during which high-energy sound waves are directed at the painful part of the plantar fascia. This technique is similar to the one used to break up kidney stones, but does not direct sufficient energy at the foot to break up the heel bone or any heel spurs. Some studies have reported that the technique relieves pain in 60% to 80% of those treated, while causing only minimal complications or side effects, which can include periodic pain in the treated area. Other studies have shown only limited benefit, and there is an overall lack of evidence to assess its effectiveness. This technique is gaining acceptance, however, and may be included in a physical therapy program. Talk with your own foot care specialist about the latest research and whether shock wave treatment is right for you. Also be aware that many health insurers do not cover this technology, so you may want to check your coverage before undergoing treatment.

Achilles' tendinitis and tendinosis

Heel pain may occur when the Achilles' tendon, which runs up the back of the heel, suffers damage, inflammation, or degeneration. With Achilles' tendinitis, the tendon becomes inflamed. A separate yet related problem, Achilles' tendinosis, occurs when the tendon actually degrades—much like a rope fraying. Because the symptoms and treatment of these two problems are virtually the same, you may not know whether you have Achilles' tendinitis or tendinosis unless you ask your doctor. Many patients have both disorders. But it's good to know, because if you develop Achilles' tendinosis, it's vital that you take steps to protect your tendon from further structural damage.

Usually, Achilles' tendinitis occurs from overuse or exertion while running (especially up and down hills, when more strain is placed on the tendon), but poorly fitting shoes may also be to blame. Women who start wearing flat shoes after years of high heels may also develop Achilles' tendinitis because the lower position of the heel stretches the Achilles' tendon to its full length.

The pain of Achilles' tendinitis is sometimes accompanied by swelling or stiffness that worsens with exercise. To prevent this problem, do warm-up stretches before you exercise (see "Limber up," page 8). Also, make sure your shoes fit properly. An athletic shoe that digs into your heel or provides little support is an invitation to trouble.

Weight gain often contributes to the development of Achilles' tendinosis. Although the tendon begins to degrade for a number of reasons, including genetic

> ### Plantar fascia–specific stretching exercise
> Sit in a chair with the one foot on the floor and the other ankle on your knee. Grasp the toes with your hand and gently pull the toes back until you feel a stretch in the sole of your foot. At the same time, gently massage the stretched plantar fascia with your other hand. Hold for 10 seconds. Repeat 10 times, three times per day.

susceptibility to such damage, extra weight adds to the strain on the tendon and accelerates the destruction.

> **SYMPTOMS OF Achilles' tendinitis and tendinosis**
> - Pain at the back of your heel
> - Pain that intensifies if you exercise
> - Possible tenderness and swelling of the heel

Treating Achilles' tendinitis and tendinosis

Treatment of both Achilles' tendinitis and Achilles' tendinosis involves a regimen known as RICE—rest, ice, compression, and elevation (see "First aid: The RICE regimen," page 22)—and nonprescription pain relievers (see Table 2, page 41). If the tendon is swollen and warm, you may benefit from an NSAID such as aspirin, ibuprofen, or naproxen for three to four weeks in order to reduce inflammation.

Once the pain and swelling are gone, try to stretch the tendon gently to strengthen it. The stretching exercises recommended for the bottom of your feet can help (see "Bottom of foot," page 8).

The plantar fascia works with the Achilles' tendon, lever-and-pulley style, to move the foot. Your foot care specialist may also prescribe heel lifts or Achilles' heel cushions to provide heel support and take pressure off the Achilles' tendons. If the pain and swelling persist, see a foot care specialist, who may prescribe physical therapy to alleviate your symptoms. In addition, a night splint can help by keeping the Achilles' tendon in a stretched position while you sleep. Don't expect immediate results. Typically, these conditions heal within six to 12 months. If the tendon has completely ruptured or torn away from the bone, you may need surgery.

Posterior heel bursitis

A bursa is a fluid-filled sac that cushions a tendon near a bone. If a bursa becomes inflamed, the painful condition is known as bursitis. The problem may develop because of an abnormal bone structure that irritates the surrounding tissues, poorly fitting shoes, or prolonged walking or running. When you feel pain at the back of your heel, it may be posterior heel bursitis. To prevent this type of bursitis, make sure that your shoes fit correctly and provide plenty of cushioning.

> **SYMPTOMS OF Posterior heel bursitis**
> - Pain at the back of your heel
> - Pain that grows worse when you stand for a long time
> - Pain that intensifies by the end of the day

Treating posterior heel bursitis

If posterior heel bursitis develops, it's generally treated much like Achilles' tendinitis and Achilles' tendinosis. Try the RICE regimen first, along with a nonprescription pain reliever. If swelling persists, you may need to take an NSAID (see Table 2) for three to four weeks to reduce inflammation. Once the pain and swelling are gone, stretch the tendon gently to strengthen it. If the pain persists, see a foot care specialist, who may suggest shoe inserts (such as heel lifts or Achilles' heel cushions) or physical therapy to alleviate your discomfort. As with other heel problems, posterior heel bursitis can take anywhere from six to 12 months to heal.

Arches that ache and flat feet

If the middle of your foot hurts, it may reflect a change in the structural integrity of your arch. In extreme cases, arches can collapse, resulting in flat feet or fallen arches. While some people are born with fallen arches, others develop the condition over time because of weakness in the tendons and soft tissues that support the arch. The major structural causes of flat feet are discussed below.

Flexible flat feet

Most children have flexible flat feet, a normal condition in which the arch flattens when pressure is applied but springs back once weight is taken off the foot. The child's arch does not fully develop until about age 10. But as many as one in five people retains flexible flat feet into adulthood, often because of an inherited tendency for loose ligaments and flexible joints. Flexible flat feet are seldom painful. In the rare cases where symptoms do occur, the person may complain of tired, aching feet after standing or walking for extended periods.

> **SYMPTOMS OF Flexible flat feet**
> - An arch that flattens under pressure
> - Aching feet after you stand or walk for a long period

Treating flexible flat feet

If you experience these symptoms, look for shoes with good arch supports or try an over-the-counter shoe insert. Although there is no best brand, you may find that one fits your foot better than another, so shop around. If your symptoms persist, talk to your foot care specialist about custom orthoses (see "Do you need orthoses?" on page 46).

Rigid flat feet

Of more concern is a condition known as rigid flat feet, in which there is no arch to your foot, even when you are sitting. About one in 100 people suffers from an inherited condition known as tarsal coalition, in which two or more foot bones are fused together, limiting flexibility and flattening the arch. Many people have no symptoms. Some will develop pain in their teens. The pain may worsen with exertion.

> **SYMPTOMS OF Rigid flat feet**
> - Lack of an arch, even when no weight is on the foot
> - Pain that may start on the outside of the foot and extend up to the ankle
> - Pain that may intensify after walking or other exercise

Treating rigid flat feet

If the flat foot is painless and doesn't interfere with walking, no treatment is required. If the symptoms are not too severe, you can treat it with a combination of shoe inserts, including arch supports or custom-made orthoses, along with an NSAID such as aspirin or ibuprofen (see Table 2, page 41). Make sure your shoes fit comfortably and aren't aggravating the pain. You may find applying ice to the area helpful when the pain flares up. Your doctor may also recommend physical therapy, a walking cast, or a brace. More severe cases require surgery either to remove the bridge that has formed between the bones or to fuse them completely. Recovery from this surgery takes time—anywhere from three to six months and sometimes longer.

Posterior tibial tendon dysfunction

The posterior tibial tendon is a large tendon that runs along the inner side of your lower leg and ankle. It attaches to the inner side of your arch and is one of the arch's main support structures. In some people, this tendon can degenerate, stretch, or tear, resulting in posterior tibial tendon dysfunction. This condition may arise from an injury, but it most commonly develops because of simple wear and tear. It can be compared to the loss of elasticity that occurs in a rubber band that has been stretched too often and too long, so that it won't bounce back after it's stretched. Similarly, your posterior tibial tendon can suffer tiny tears and degradation over time, compromising its elasticity.

Early on, you'll feel pain along the inner side of the ankle and arch. Since the tendon supports the arch, you may develop a flat foot that, over time, may become rigid. Eventually the pain may extend to the outer side of your foot and ankle, and arthritis may develop.

Women who have worn high heels for extended periods may be most at risk for this condition because their Achilles' tendons have likely shortened and tightened. The other tendons and ligaments in the area try to compensate, but with time may also experience wear and tear. As they break down, arch support suffers.

> SYMPTOMS OF **Posterior tibial tendon dysfunction**
> - Pain and weakness in the tendon that runs along the inner side of the ankle
> - Pain in the arch
> - Possible development of flat feet (flexible at first)
> - Additional symptoms developing over time, including pain on the outer side of the foot or ankle, rigid flat feet, or impaired walking

Treating posterior tibial tendon dysfunction

The earlier you treat this condition, the more likely you are to avoid surgery. So, if you have symptoms of posterior tibial tendon dysfunction, it is important to see a doctor for a diagnosis. Initial treatment may consist of NSAIDs to reduce pain and inflammation (see Table 2) and custom-made orthoses, braces, or both to support the arch. Your doctor may also recommend gentle exercises so that you can stretch the Achilles' tendon and build strength in the muscles that support the foot.

The four stages of posterior tibial tendon dysfunction

Stage I: Inflammation occurs in the posterior tibial tendon, but the tendon remains strong and there is no change to the arch of the foot.

Stage II: The tendon loses strength as a result of degeneration; the arch becomes partially flattened, but there are no arthritic changes in the foot. However, pain spreads sideways.

Stage III: The posterior tibial tendon is torn and can no longer hold the arch, which collapses entirely. Arthritic changes occur in the hindfoot.

Stage IV: The ankle joint becomes arthritic.

Studies show that nonsurgical methods are effective in managing this condition when caught in its early stages, even over the long term (see "The four stages of posterior tibial tendon dysfunction," above).

One study of 32 patients with stage II posterior tibial tendon dysfunction who were treated with an ankle-foot orthosis found that after seven to 10 years, 70% of the patients were brace-free and avoided surgery, while five patients (15%) still wore a brace and another five patients (15%) went on to have surgery. Another study of 36 adults in stage I or II of the condition found that a program of stretching and orthosis-wearing improved the condition over all, and that certain resistance exercises further reduced pain and improved perception of function.

If your symptoms persist or your condition is advanced, surgery may be necessary. Several different types of surgery are used to treat posterior tibial tendon dysfunction. The most commonly used procedures include an osteotomy of the heel bone (calcaneus), which involves cutting and shifting the bone to realign the position of the foot, and a tendon transfer, in which the posterior tibial tendon is repaired using fibers from another tendon. The exact procedure used will depend on the severity of your symptoms and whether your arch has collapsed.

Tormented toes

Your toes are small compared with the rest of your body, yet they perform a number of vital functions. Toes increase the stability, balance, and strength of the entire foot. Toe deformities can result from a problem in another part of the foot or even further up in the leg. Several common toe deformities are discussed below. People with diabetes are susceptible to toe problems because the nerve and circulatory impairment that accompanies this disease can affect the feet.

This section describes structural toe problems. Conditions relating to the skin of the toes, such as corns, ingrown toenails, and foot fungus, are discussed later (see "Skin and toenail problems," page 24).

Bunions and bunionettes

Bunions are among the most common causes of painful toes. They plague more than half of all American women, according to the American Academy of Orthopaedic Surgeons, but only a quarter of men. They are twice as common among people over age 60, compared with younger adults. A bunion isn't a growth, but rather a misalignment of the bones in the foot. This occurs when the metatarsophalangeal joint and the first metatarsal of the toe deviate away from the other metatarsal bones, causing the big toe to turn inward, bending toward (or even under) the other toes. The medical term for bunion—hallux valgus deformity—is a more literal description of the condition. *Hallux* is Latin for big toe, and *valgus* is Latin for misalignment. A bunionette is a similar condition affecting the base of the small fifth toe and is sometimes called a "tailor's bunion," because tailors once sat cross-legged all day, with the outer sides of their feet rubbing on the ground.

Bunions and bunionettes can result from heredity, arthritis, or misalignment of the foot. But the most frequent cause is the prolonged wearing of shoes that squeeze the toes into pointy or narrow toe boxes, forcing the toes to fold over one another to fit in. Over time, a bunion or bunionette develops. Small surprise, then, that nine out of 10 bunions occur in women.

Neither condition may cause any pain at first, but you might notice that you have developed a bump on the side of your foot and that it's harder to put on tight shoes. In time, a bunion or bunionette can become extremely painful.

Treating bunions and bunionettes

You may be able to prevent bunions and bunionettes from developing—or keep them from getting worse—by wearing shoes that provide sufficient room in the toe boxes. Look for shoes with blunt toes rather than pointy ones, and allow for about a quarter-inch to a half-inch of space between your longest toe and the front of the shoe.

If you've already developed a bunion or bunionette, you can help alleviate the pain by padding the protuberance with felt, moleskin, or a donut-shaped pad. Another helpful aid is a shoe stretcher with a special plastic plug that can be placed in the shoe to stretch the bunion/bunionette area, thereby relieving the pressure on your foot at that point. Orthoses can redistribute your weight so the bunion doesn't constantly rub against your shoe. A recent article in the *Journal of the American Academy of Orthopedic Surgery* suggested that orthoses can play an important role in the nonsurgical management of several foot conditions, including those caused by arthritis, as is sometimes the case with bunions and bunionettes.

> ▶ SYMPTOMS OF **Bunions and bunionettes**
>
> - Bony protuberance at base of big toe (for bunion) or fifth toe (for bunionette)
> - Pain, especially when wearing shoes that press against the bump

FOOT FACT for women

As many as seven in 10 American women have developed a bunion, hammertoe, or other disabling foot condition, usually as a result of wearing improperly fitting shoes.

Mild and moderate bunions may not hurt, but severe bunions—in which the protuberance is large and the big toe slants noticeably toward the others—usually do. Only a doctor can determine the severity of your bunion, but if it hurts, take action. To deal with pain, especially when the bunion or bunionette is inflamed, try NSAID pain relievers (see Table 2, page 41). Hot and cold compresses may also help. If these steps don't work, and you are still experiencing significant pain that interferes with daily activities, you may need to consider surgery to restore the toe to its normal position. Surgery is a major step that does not always eliminate all symptoms and will require you to stay off your foot for six to 12 weeks.

If your doctor recommends surgery, the specific procedure will depend on the severity of your condition. Several procedures are available. To treat mild bunions, for example, the surgeon might use the modified McBride procedure by shaving the enlarged portion of the bone and realigning the muscles, tendons, and ligaments. Recovery from this type of surgery typically takes at least six weeks. For moderate misalignments, the surgeon may use the chevron procedure to cut the bone close to the metatarsal head and then shift it back into its proper position. In this case, recovery takes about six to 12 weeks, during which you may be advised not to walk on your foot. To correct severe bunions, a cut must be made further down the metatarsal bone (see Figure 4). The surgeon may keep the bones in position with pins, screws, or plates. Recovery from this procedure, known as a proximal osteotomy, takes at least three months.

The decision to have surgery should be made very carefully. Some people still experience residual symptoms after undergoing surgery, which makes sense considering that the procedure moves muscles, ligaments, and bones that have been accustomed to being in the same place for your entire life. Moving them to a new position can, in itself, cause pain in some people.

Surgery to correct a moderate to severe bunion will require you to stop driving for about six weeks. One study found that patients were able to drive safely six weeks following bunion surgery, indicating that they had low pain levels. The study, published in 2008 in the *Journal of Bone and Joint Surgery*, also found that emergency brake time response in patients who underwent surgery was similar to that of healthy individuals just six weeks after the procedure. However, if the surgery is performed to correct a moderate to severe bunion on the right foot, you risk reinjuring your foot if you resume driving before the six-week mark, the study found.

During recovery from bunion surgery, you may have to wear a bandage and special shoe—or possibly a cast in more severe cases. The special shoe or cast will protect your foot, allowing it to heal, while enabling you to walk on your heel. During recovery, your muscles and other soft tissues will atrophy, so

Figure 4 Surgical correction of a bunion

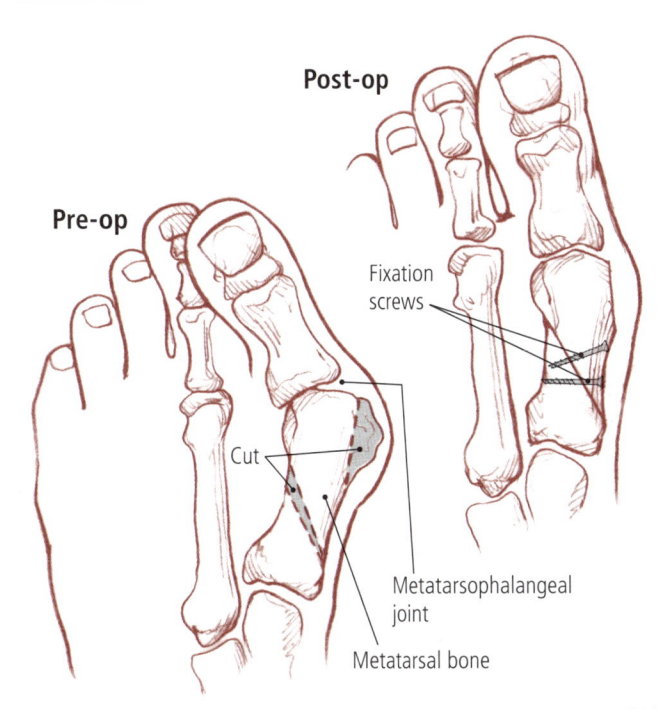

© Harriet Greenfield

The procedure illustrated above, known as a proximal osteotomy, is used to correct a severe bunion. First, the surgeon cuts away a portion of the bunion at the head of the metatarsal bone. Next, he or she removes a pie-shaped segment from the lower portion of the same bone, allowing for realignment of the metatarsophalangeal joint. Two pins or screws fasten the bone segments.

after the postoperative shoe or cast is removed, you may have to do exercises to regain your strength and flexibility. It may take as long as six months to recover fully (to the point where you can do strenuous activities). Similar surgical procedures can be performed for bunionettes, and the recovery time is usually somewhat shorter.

Hammertoe

Another cause of toe pain is a hammertoe, a deformity that develops when tendons and ligaments in the toe contract, causing the toe to bend over and curl up—resembling a hammer. The top of your toe may then rub against your shoe, causing irritation, corns, calluses, or even bursitis. The problem usually develops in the second toe, often because a bunion has formed in the big toe, forcing it inward and displacing the second toe. Shoes with narrow toe boxes, which compress the toes, increase the risk for a hammertoe. Women are four times as likely as men to develop hammertoe because they more often wear narrow shoes. In addition, shoes such as clogs, flip-flops, and sandals that require your toes to grip in order to keep the shoe on can increase your risk of developing hammertoes.

Two closely related conditions—mallet toe (where the toe is bent only at the tip) and claw toe (where the toe is more severely contracted at all three joints)—reflect the same basic problem. The tendency to develop hammertoe, claw toe, or mallet toe runs in families. These problems may also develop as a secondary effect of an underlying disorder, such as arthritis. But for most people, the best way to prevent these deformities is to wear shoes that provide enough room for your toes.

Treating hammertoe and similar conditions

Usually, hammertoes are flexible at first. Apply pressure to the toe, and it will flatten back down. In such cases, you can relieve irritation by making a crest pad (out of moleskin or foam) so when you put on your shoe, the top of the shoe will press down on the crest pad and keep the toe down for as long as you have the shoe on. Still, once a hammertoe or other toe deformity has developed, no amount of "retraining" will make it lie flat permanently. In time, even if you wear a crest pad, a hammertoe can become rigid and may become more painful and inflamed.

You can relieve hammertoe pain and inflammation by applying ice or cold compresses or by soaking your foot in warm water. Exercising the toe may help as well. If it doesn't help, purchase a splint to provide support, a shoe stretcher to provide more room, or an insert to redistribute your weight and ease pressure on the affected toe. For severe cases, surgery may be necessary. For flexible hammertoe, a surgeon may do a tendon transfer—relocating a tendon from underneath the toe to restore the toe to its normal position. For rigid hammertoe, the surgeon will most likely have to remove a part of the bone.

Osteoarthritis

Arthritis is a disease that affects joints—and each foot has 33 of them! So it should come as no surprise that your feet are especially susceptible. Osteoarthritis is characterized by pain and stiffness early in the morning, which diminishes as you move about but gradually returns later in the day. As you try to compensate for the pain, your gait may become abnormal, and you may even limp. Rest may help alleviate the symptoms.

There are about 100 types of arthritis, but osteoarthritis and gout (see next section) are two types that commonly affect the feet. Although any part of the foot can suffer, toes are most frequently affected. One of the most common ailments is hallux rigidus, which involves the loss of flexibility in the big toe due to osteoarthritis in the metatarsophalangeal joint.

Osteoarthritis is caused by wear and tear or injury and generally develops over time. It involves the gradual erosion of a joint's surrounding cartilage, leaving less cushioning between bones, which in turn causes pain and sometimes inflammation. Since the feet sup-

> ▶ SYMPTOMS OF **Hammertoe**
>
> - Bending and curling of a toe—usually the second toe, but possibly any of the three middle toes—so its shape resembles a hammer
> - With time, pain and irritation on the top of the toe

> **SYMPTOMS OF Osteoarthritis**
>
> - Pain in the morning that gradually recedes but returns at the end of the day
> - Pain that is alleviated by resting the affected joint
> - Stiffness in the affected joint

port most of the body's weight, they are especially susceptible. Obesity can add to the problem by putting more pressure on joints. A 2008 government study, one of the largest ever to monitor the onset of osteoarthritis, found that obese people had the highest risk for developing osteoarthritis—which is why maintaining a healthy weight is so important. A severe foot injury or a history of previous injuries (as from playing sports) can also make the feet more susceptible to osteoarthritis.

Does high-impact, repetitive exercise such as running, aerobics, dancing, or playing sports contribute to osteoarthritis? The jury is still out on this question. On the one hand, your joints take a real pounding, as every heel strike occurs at a force of three or four times your body's weight, possibly causing damage over time. On the other hand, experts believe that high-impact exercise has a protective effect on the joints, thickening cartilage that surrounds them and also keeping body weight down.

Treating osteoarthritis

Stretching and strengthening exercises can help relieve pain by maintaining joint flexibility and by conditioning the muscles that support the arthritic joint. Gentle stretching exercises, such as those in the Special Section of this report (see page 6), can help loosen your joints, keeping them limber and easing pressure on the surrounding cartilage. You can also reduce pain and any inflammation with hot and cold packs, NSAIDs, or a COX-2 inhibitor such as celecoxib (Celebrex). These medications have a variety of side effects, so it is important to discuss your personal health risks with your doctor when considering their long-term use (see Table 2, page 41). Your doctor may also recommend orthoses to adjust your walking gait in a way that will take pressure off aching joints.

If these strategies don't alleviate your arthritis pain, surgery to repair or replace damaged joints may be necessary. One thing to be aware of: you may have arthritis that shows up in an x-ray and not have any pain or other symptoms. If so, that's fine. On the other hand, your x-ray may reveal little in the way of structural damage even if you are experiencing pain severe enough to interfere with your ability to walk. If you have significant pain, see a foot care specialist. Treatment decisions are based on symptoms, not x-ray evidence.

To help protect your feet from injury—which can lead to osteoarthritis—wear well-fitting, well-built shoes with cushioned soles (see "What to look for in a shoe," page 45) and check with a podiatrist or orthopedist about whether you can benefit from an orthotic insert, especially if you run or do other sports. There's no foolproof way to prevent osteoarthritis, because cartilage erosion progresses with age. But if you start noticing joint pain in your feet, you may be able to slow the progress of the disease by wearing appropriate footwear and orthoses, either purchased over the counter or, if needed, custom made.

Gout

This condition is the most common form of inflammatory arthritis in men, and its incidence has increased since the late 1980s. Gout causes arthritic symptoms when uric acid, a normal byproduct of digestion, accumulates in the joints. A person with gout either makes too much uric acid or cannot excrete it properly. As a result, the uric acid forms crystals that settle in the joints and cause inflammation, sudden jabs of pain, soreness, redness, and swelling. In the foot, gout most often affects the joint at the base of the big toe.

Although everyone makes uric acid naturally, levels of this compound can increase when you eat certain foods that contain substances known as purines, such as organ meats, sardines, and some shellfish (see "Purines in food," page 20). Purines increase pro-

> **SYMPTOMS OF Gout**
>
> - Jolts of pain in the affected joint
> - Possible inflammation in the joint
> - Increase in symptoms after eating some foods

duction of lactate, which competes with uric acid for excretion. Gout affects men more frequently than women, probably because men have higher uric acid levels than women. That changes at menopause, however, which explains why men tend to develop gout between ages 30 and 50, while women are more likely to develop it after age 50.

Treating gout

To treat an attack of gout, your doctor will usually begin by prescribing an NSAID (see Table 2, page 41). Avoid aspirin, as it may raise uric acid levels. If you cannot tolerate NSAIDs or if they do not help, your doctor may suggest a corticosteroid, such as prednisone, to reduce inflammation. Corticosteroids may be taken orally; less frequently, they are injected directly into the affected joint (usually numbed ahead of time with a nerve block). Another option is an injection of adrenocorticotrophic hormone, a compound that directs your adrenal gland to make more cortisone. Although the medication colchicine may be given in pill form, it tends to cause unpleasant side effects (nausea, vomiting, cramps, and diarrhea). Rarely, people may take drugs to lower uric acid levels in their blood. These include probenecid (Benemid, Probalan) to increase urinary excretion of uric acid, and allopurinol (Zyloprim) and febuxostat (Uloric) to reduce the body's production of uric acid. Allopurinol is a good choice for most people, as it is available as a generic and therefore far less expensive. But for people who are allergic to allopurinol or cannot tolerate it, febuxostat might be a better alternative.

Sesamoid pain

Beneath the base of your big toe, in the ball of your foot, are two small bones called the sesamoids. They function much like pulleys, facilitating movement of the big toe. But with too much stress, they can become irritated and inflamed—a condition known as sesamoiditis—and may even fracture. The best way to avoid the problem is to wear shoes with proper support and cushioning, especially for high-impact sports such as tennis or running.

> **SYMPTOMS OF Sesamoid pain**
> - Pain in the ball of the foot, beneath the big toe
> - Swelling in the ball of the foot

Treating sesamoid pain

If this problem develops, applying ice to the area helps relieve pain and inflammation. You may have to cushion the area to relieve pressure on the bones—with soft over-the-counter shoe inserts or orthoses with padding—until the inflammation subsides, often in about two to three months. Rest and an NSAID pain reliever (see Table 2, page 41) can also help. If the pain persists for more than a few weeks, see a foot care specialist, who will x-ray the area to assess the bones and tailor your treatment program to the diagnosis.

Purines in food

Foods with high purine content
People with gout should avoid eating these foods:

- anchovies
- bouillon
- brains
- broth
- consommé
- goose
- gravy
- heart
- herring
- kidney
- lentils
- liver
- mackerel
- meat extracts
- mincemeat
- mussels
- partridge
- roe
- sardines
- scallops
- sweetbreads
- yeast

Foods with moderate purine content
People with gout should limit themselves to no more than one serving per day of these foods. A serving is 3.5 ounces (100 grams) of meat or fish or one-half cup of vegetables.

- asparagus
- beans
- cauliflower
- fish
- meat
- mushrooms
- oatmeal
- dried peas
- poultry
- shellfish
- spinach

Missteps and mishaps: Foot injuries

Who hasn't misjudged a curb and stumbled, or stubbed a toe on a piece of furniture? Such accidents can cause a fracture or sprain. Here are a few common foot injuries and how to treat them.

Fractures

Broken bones can take the form of a clean break, chipped bones, or stress fractures—incomplete hairline cracks that result from repetitive, low-impact stress (see "Stress fractures," below). The bone-thinning disease, osteoporosis, can contribute to fractures, so make sure to get the Recommended Dietary Allowance (RDA) of vitamin D and calcium to protect your bone health. The RDA for vitamin D is 600 IU for most adults and 800 IU for people over age 70. The RDA for calcium is 1,000 milligrams for adults up to age 50 and 1,200 for adults 50 and over. Symptoms of fractures include pain, bruising, and an inability to put weight on the foot.

All fractures require immediate attention. An untreated fracture might not heal properly and could result in deformity, persistent pain, or both. If you suspect that you've fractured your foot, have it looked at right away. Although any bone in the foot can break, fractures occur most frequently in the toes (phalanges), when a person stubs the toe or drops something on it. The metatarsals—the long, thin bones that lead from the toes to the arch—are likewise common fracture sites. Metatarsal injuries typically occur if something is dropped on the foot or if it's forcefully twisted.

How do you know if you've broken a bone in your foot? You'll need an x-ray to tell for sure, but to complicate matters, bones break in many different ways, and subtle damage, such as a hairline fracture, can be difficult to detect. It can take two weeks for evidence of the body's attempt to heal a bone fracture to show up as an abnormality on an x-ray. So it's important to pay attention to symptoms. One warning sign of a fracture is difficulty in walking after an injury. Don't be fooled, however. It's sometimes possible to walk on a broken foot, so check to see whether you have any pain or tenderness directly over the bone when you touch it lightly. Such focal pain may indicate a fracture, especially if it persists after you've rested briefly and followed the RICE regimen (see page 22). Your best bet, if you have any doubts, is to get an x-ray, which may reveal whether you've broken a bone and, if so, whether it needs to be realigned. If an initial x-ray does not reveal a fracture, but the pain persists for more than 10 to 14 days, ask for a follow-up x-ray immediately to make sure a bone is not broken.

Treating a foot fracture

Treatment generally consists of protecting the fractured bone as it heals by wearing a special hard-soled shoe or a plastic-and-foam fracture boot. You may or may not be able to walk, depending on the nature and location of the fracture. If you've broken just your toe, your doctor may simply "buddy tape" it to an adjacent toe to help stabilize it while it heals. For larger breaks, your doctor may prescribe a splint or even a cast. If fragments of bone were significantly displaced, the fracture may require surgery. Healing time varies and may be anywhere from two to 12 weeks.

Stress fractures

Stress fractures are hairline cracks in a bone. In young people, these can develop as the result of overexertion or prolonged high-impact exercise, such as running

---

▶ SYMPTOMS OF **Foot fracture**

- Pain directly over a bone
- Pain and swelling that persist even after the RICE regimen
- Inability to walk on the affected foot

or tennis. But they may also occur in middle-aged or elderly people, especially women, who experience a reduction in bone density (osteopenia) or the more severe condition known as osteoporosis. People with such conditions may develop stress fractures even as a result of normal daily activities, such as walking. In the feet, stress fractures most often occur in the metatarsal bones (the long bones leading to the toes), but they can also occur in the heel.

The best way to prevent a stress fracture is to avoid sudden increases in activity or exercise by gradually building up your exercise regimen. Wear well-cushioned shoes to reduce the impact on your feet. Warm up before you exercise, because limber muscles allow better joint motion and flexibility, which in turn helps cushion the impact on your bones. Try some exercises for foot fitness (see page 8).

Treating a stress fracture

If you think you have a stress fracture, see your doctor. He or she will probably order an x-ray. But because stress fractures don't always show up in x-rays, your doctor may have to diagnose the condition by feeling the area or ordering other tests such as a bone scan or an MRI. Whatever you do, don't continue exercising if you have point tenderness (localized pain over a bone). You might break it completely.

If you do have a stress fracture, your doctor will probably recommend rest and some type of immobilizing device, such as a special hard-soled shoe or a fracture boot. Researchers are looking at whether osteoporosis medications such as teriparatide (Forteo) can be used to help stress fractures heal. Typically, stress fractures heal within four to six weeks.

> **SYMPTOMS OF Stress fracture**
>
> - Point tenderness—pain when you press on a bone
> - Possible redness and swelling
> - Pain that develops after you increase your activity level or, if you are middle-aged or older, with your normal activity level

Sprains

A foot sprain involves tearing a ligament, a fibrous structure that connects one bone to another. One common type of foot sprain is a midfoot sprain. It can occur when you stumble or fall and your foot twists oddly, or when you sustain a sudden impact to the middle of your foot, such as during an auto accident or a fall from a high place.

Another common sprain affects the big toe. It usually occurs at the metatarsophalangeal joint, and it's also known as "turf toe" because it often affects football players who compete on unforgiving artificial turf. However, anyone can experience turf toe, which occurs when the big toe is bent too far back toward the ankle. Whatever the cause, a sprain around this joint will cause pain, swelling, tenderness, and possibly bruising.

The best way to avoid sprains is by wearing sturdy shoes with thick soles, such as good walking, running, or cross-training shoes, which will help protect vulnerable areas of your foot. You can also help prevent strains by doing exercises for foot fitness and by warming up before exercising.

> **First aid: The RICE regimen**
>
> If you injure your foot in some way, remember the acronym **RICE**. Four simple steps will help limit pain and additional damage:
>
> **Rest.** Take the pressure off your injured foot by reducing your activity and sitting or lying down.
>
> **Ice.** To reduce inflammation, apply ice to the injury. You can crush the ice or wrap it in a towel to be more comfortable. Put the ice in a plastic bag so it doesn't soak your clothing or furniture as it melts. You can also use an ice pack, a chemical cold pack, or even a bag of frozen peas for this purpose.
>
> **Compression.** Wrap an elastic compression bandage around the injured area to provide support and reduce swelling. Wrap it snugly, but not tightly enough to impede the circulation of blood. If your toes turn white or purple, if they feel numb, or if you get a pins-and-needles feeling, loosen the bandage.
>
> **Elevation.** To reduce inflammation and pain, prop your foot on a pillow or on the arm of a sofa—anywhere it will be raised above your waist level.

> SYMPTOMS OF **Sprain**
> - Pain accompanied by swelling and tenderness
> - Pain that develops after the entire foot or a particular joint is twisted or bent at an odd angle

Treating a sprain

If you do sustain a sprain, follow the RICE regimen and take an NSAID for one to four weeks (depending on the severity of your sprain) to alleviate the pain and inflammation (see Table 2, page 41).

If you're unable to bear weight on the injured foot, see a doctor who can check for a possible fracture. More severe sprains may require splinting or even a cast. A sprain can take anywhere from a few days to several months to heal, depending on its severity and location. Often recuperation will involve a brief period of staying off the injured foot.

Skin and toenail problems

Your skin and toenails reveal a lot about your overall health and can provide the first sign of a systemic disease. For instance, nails that are rounded inward like spoons, rather than outward, may indicate a severe iron deficiency. Nails that are pitted and thick are a sign of psoriasis. If you notice any abnormality in the shape or color of your toenails, ask your foot care specialist about it.

Many treatments are available for skin and toenail conditions, by prescription or over the counter. Drugstores carry a host of remedies for corns, calluses, fungal infections, and warts. Some of these are worth trying; others should only be used with caution. The challenge is to know when to do something on your own and when to consult a doctor or foot care specialist. The following are major problems involving the nails and skin and options for treating them.

Ingrown toenails

An ingrown toenail is one of the most common sources of foot pain. It can be a serious problem for anyone with diabetes or circulatory difficulties (see "Diabetes," page 33, and "Vascular problems and cold feet," page 37).

An ingrown toenail develops when the side of the nail digs into the skin. This can lead to pain, irritation, swelling, and redness. The big toe is most often affected, although no toe is immune. The problem usually develops because the nails have not been trimmed properly. Overly tight shoes may also be a factor. Some people have an inherited tendency to develop the problem.

The easiest way to prevent an ingrown toenail is to cut your nails straight across, rather than rounding off the corners (as you would with your fingernails). Use a toenail clipper (which is wider and larger than a fingernail clipper) or, if you use scissors, cut the nail in several short movements. Also, clean under your nails regularly. Wear shoes that provide enough room at the toes, and wear stockings or socks that allow your toes to move freely.

> **SYMPTOMS OF Ingrown toenail**
> - Pain in the toe that increases when it is pressed
> - A nail edge that digs into the side of the toe
> - A toe that's red or warm to the touch

Treating ingrown toenails

You can treat this problem at home, unless you have diabetes. If you have diabetes and have an ingrown toenail, you should see your doctor or foot care specialist immediately. Otherwise, if the problem is minor (the toe is irritated and red, but not overwhelmingly painful), soak your feet in warm water to soften the nail, then cut the part of the nail that is pressing against the skin. Trim gently, not aggressively, or you may hurt yourself.

Once that part of the nail is removed, apply an over-the-counter topical antibiotic. Wear open-toed sandals or roomy shoes to reduce pressure on the toe. If your toe isn't better in three to five days, see a foot care specialist. Your toe may be infected, and you may need to start oral antibiotics and have the ingrown portion of the nail removed. Once the problem is successfully treated, allow the nail to grow out to the point where you can trim it straight across, and avoid wearing shoes with narrow toes.

Ingrown toenails can become chronic, occurring over and over again. If so, your doctor may

> **FOOT FACTS**
> - Nails grow faster in summer than in winter.
> - Men's nails generally grow faster than women's.

decide to remove the part of the nail that's been causing the problem. This office procedure can be done with chemicals rather than with a scalpel, so you can avoid a trip to the operating room. Even with treatment, this condition can cause permanent changes to the nail bed.

Blisters

Chances are you've suffered a blister at some point in your life, perhaps because you were trying to break in a new pair of shoes or because your feet swelled on a hot day and rubbed against your shoes. Blisters are fluid-filled sacs that develop between the top layers of skin after prolonged pressure or rubbing, which causes irritation. Blisters occur most often on the heel, the toes, or the ball of the foot. A friction blister contains clear fluid; a blood blister develops when small blood vessels are damaged and leak. A blister will hurt if you touch it, and it may break unless you take steps to bandage and protect it.

The best way to prevent blisters is to wear shoes that fit comfortably—not so tight as to cause continuous pressure, and not so loose that they slide up and down your heel when you walk. Also, make sure your feet remain dry during the day, since moist feet tend to "stick" to the shoe and worsen rubbing. Wear socks or stockings to pad the skin and minimize any friction as you walk. If you are prone to blisters or know that particular shoes cause problems, use petroleum jelly to lubricate the skin in a problem area, or foot powder to keep your feet dry. You can also protect the skin at problem spots using bandages or moleskin.

> ▶ SYMPTOMS OF **Blister**
> - Soft, fluid-filled bubble of skin at a part of the foot exposed to friction
> - Fluid that is usually clear, but may contain traces of blood

Treating blisters

If a blister develops, don't pop it. The skin provides a natural defense against infection. A blister should drain on its own in a few days, as a new layer of skin forms underneath the fluid. The outer layer will eventually peel away. To prevent the blister from popping, place a bandage over it, or—for large blisters—create a donut cushion by cutting a hole in a piece of moleskin or felt. If the blister breaks anyway, clean and dry the area and use an antibiotic ointment before covering it with a sterile bandage. If you have diabetes or a circulatory problem, it may take longer for the blister to heal on its own, and you'll be more likely to develop an infection. Consult a doctor or foot care specialist.

If you have a blister so large and painful that it interferes with walking, seek medical help. Also seek help if you notice that the fluid in the blister is not clear but looks more like pus, or if you develop a fever. These are signs of infection. If you have a blister that itches, or what appears to be a rash of blisters spreading across your foot, the problem may be athlete's foot or some other disorder. In any of these situations, consult your doctor or foot care specialist.

Calluses and corns

Many people have calluses or corns, or both. They appear as areas of hardened, sometimes yellow skin on pressure points or around bony areas of the foot. Calluses and corns develop to protect the foot from damage. The usual culprit is a poorly fitting shoe, but some people have inherited bone structure or gait patterns that make them more susceptible. Injuries that damage the bone structure may also lead to the development of corns and calluses.

What's the difference between the two? A big difference is location. Calluses usually form on the bottom of the feet; corns form on top, usually around the toes (see Figure 5). Calluses may develop in response to pressure in an area that doesn't have natural fat pads for protection. Or they may develop in feet that have some type of structural aberration, such as high arches or tight muscles or tendons in the heel area, which put extra strain on a bone. In any event, calluses usually develop after prolonged wear and tear or rubbing against a shoe. Corns more often develop because of irritation caused by tight shoes. Calluses generally consist of a broad area of thickened skin; corns may have a dense knot of skin in the center, indicating where most of the pressure is. "Hard" corns generally develop on the top or sides of toes, and "soft" corns in between toes.

At first, you may not notice a corn or callus. But if whatever is causing the irritation continues, the corn or callus may become larger and cause discomfort and even pain. Corns tend to grow with time unless the pressure (such as a tight shoe) is removed. If the pressure continues, a corn may become painful and eventually interfere with walking. Calluses are often painless, but those that form because of some structural problem, such as a hammertoe or a bone misalignment, can progress to the point of causing pain and interfering with your ability to walk. The area around both corns and calluses can also become discolored, turning brown, red, or black.

To prevent calluses and corns from developing, be sure to wear shoes that fit comfortably, provide cushioning in the sole, and leave enough room at the toes.

Figure 5 Distinguishing a corn from a callus

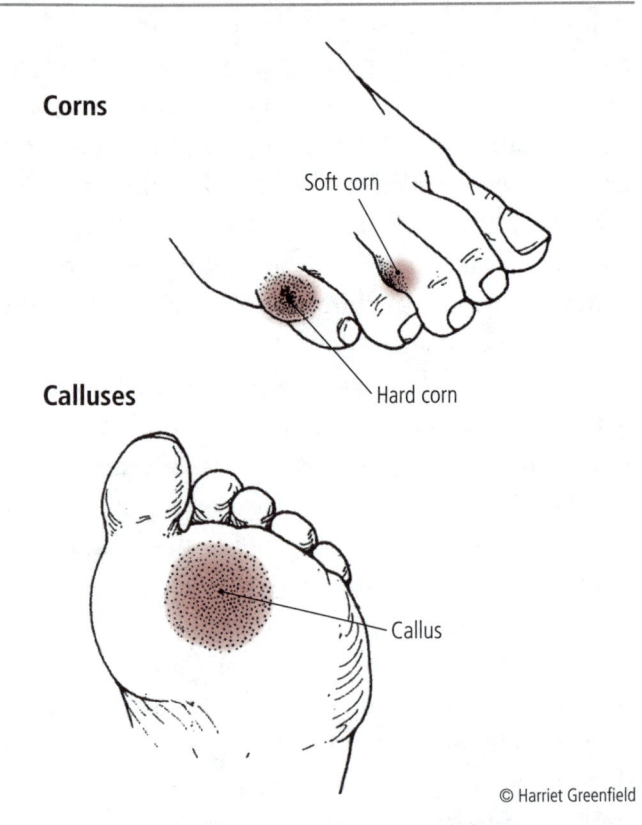

Corns
- Soft corn
- Hard corn

Calluses
- Callus

© Harriet Greenfield

Excessive pressure and friction on one area of the foot cause skin cells to multiply and then die, forming a thickened area of skin known as a corn or a callus, depending on its location. Corns form on or between toes; calluses form on the bottom of the feet.

▶ SYMPTOMS OF Calluses and corns

Calluses
- Hard, dead layer of skin, usually yellowish and flat, usually on the bottom of the foot

Corns
- Pain
- Hard, dead layer of skin, usually around the toes
- Sometimes a dense knot of skin in the center of the hardened area

Avoid pointy shoes that squeeze your toes together and high heels that shift your weight forward onto your toes. Also, wear socks or stockings to cushion your feet and reduce friction. You can add extra cushioning to shoes by inserting a padded insole. Foot powder, which will keep your feet dry, also reduces friction.

Treating calluses and corns

If you are prone to corns or calluses, cushion the affected area with moleskin to relieve pressure, and consider getting shoes with wider toe boxes. You can also make a donut with moleskin, lamb's wool, felt, or foam. Many pharmacies sell over-the-counter products to cushion corns and calluses, which you may find helpful. You may want to try custom orthoses that will redistribute your weight and take pressure off the affected areas. Another option is to use a shoe stretcher to provide more space around the corn or callus.

Better-fitting shoes will reduce the irritation that caused the problem in the first place, and over time, the corns or calluses will shrink on their own. But don't expect overnight results; the process will take weeks or even months. If you can't wait that long, you can treat the problem on your own in most cases. An important exception is if you have diabetes, peripheral neuropathy, or some other circulatory problem. In that case, never try to treat a corn or callus yourself, or you may develop an infection.

Otherwise, you can use a pumice stone, which will gently remove the top layers of skin. Soak your feet in warm water first, to soften the corn or callus. Dry your feet, then rub the pumice stone gently over the corn or callus. Afterward, moisturize the area with skin lotion. The key word is gentle; don't overdo it, or you could hurt your skin. Pharmacies sell various chemical peels and acid disks, but use such products with caution; most of them contain salicylic acid, which can damage healthy tissue unless you follow the instructions exactly. Some foot care specialists advise against using these products at all.

For larger corns and calluses, consult a foot care specialist, who will shave away some of the thickened skin. Although some pedicurists may offer to remove corns and calluses, it's safer to seek help from a trained medical specialist. (In fact, some states do not allow pedicurists to use sharp instruments or blades on the foot.) In some instances, surgery may be necessary to correct an underlying problem of bone structure, especially if you suffer from recurrent corns and calluses.

Toenail fungus

Fungal nails are fairly common, but they can go undetected for years because the initial symptoms are so subtle. The problem, known medically as onychomycosis, develops when a fungus infects the area under the surface of a toenail. There are many types of fungal infections, which are believed to affect 3% to 5% of people in the United States at any given time. Only about one in four of these people seeks help. Podiatrists, however, think these estimates are far too low, and that the percentage affected is even higher. A 2008 study that tracked the most common skin and nail fungal infections around the globe found that in the past several decades, these infections have increased steadily, and now affect more than 20% to 25% of the world's population.

The risk of developing fungal nails increases with age. About half of all Americans will have at least one affected toenail by the time they reach age 70. People with diabetes or circulation problems are more prone to develop any type of infection, including nail fungus, and anyone with an impaired immune system or a history of athlete's foot may likewise be at greater risk.

The moist, dark environment inside your shoes provides a perfect habitat for fungi. These simple plantlike organisms don't require sunlight. They also thrive on keratin, one of the proteins in toe-

> **SYMPTOMS OF Nail fungus**
>
> - Flecks of white across the nail (early sign)
> - Yellowish-brown stain on the nail
> - Flecks of green, white, or black on the nail
> - Odor
> - A nail that becomes thick and hard to cut, or that separates from the toe bed

nails. Fungi are common, so it's easy to come in contact with them. Infections are normally spread in damp areas where many people congregate—such as swimming pools and gyms, or even the shower or tub in your own home, if someone who uses it has the problem.

If a toenail becomes infected with a fungus, you may not realize it at first. A scattering of white spots may appear across the nail. This should not be confused with the occasional white lines and crescents that can develop in healthy nails. With time, the toenail becomes thicker and a yellowish-brown stain clouds the nail. White, green, and black flecks may also appear. The toes may smell. Untreated, the infection can spread to other toes and may result in numbness, tingling, pain, and nails so thick that they are difficult to cut. The end of the nail may separate from the bed underneath, and the condition may become so painful that you have trouble walking.

To prevent fungal infection, avoid walking barefoot in heavily trafficked public areas, like locker rooms or swimming pool areas. (Wear sandals or "shower shoes" when you are there.) Practice good hygiene: wash your feet daily with soap and water and dry them thoroughly, especially between the toes. Put on a pair of clean socks every day, and change them more often if you sweat a lot or get your feet wet.

Some types of socks and hose trap moisture, which encourages fungal growth. Natural fibers such as cotton absorb moisture efficiently in clothing exposed continually to the air, but when it comes to socks, there's no place for the moisture to go because the feet are encased in shoes. Cotton's wonderful absorbent quality suddenly becomes a disadvantage, and your feet may feel sweaty and damp, especially after exercising. Synthetic materials that are designed to "wick" away moisture, allowing it to evacuate up the leg, are often the best choice. Most socks today are a blend of 80% cotton with 20% synthetic fiber (such as polyester or acrylic), although some are entirely synthetic, the better choice. Wool socks can keep your feet warmer, but may cause them to perspire excessively, which encourages fungal growth.

Women may also want to reconsider using toenail polish, because it prevents moisture in the nail bed from evaporating through the nail. Make sure your toes are completely dry before applying nail polish, and always disinfect pedicure tools—even if they are your own (see "Pedicure precautions," page 31). Tight shoes that do not allow toes to "breathe" further aggravate the problem and can encourage fungal growth.

Treating nail fungus

Treatment will depend on the severity of your fungal infection. If you have a mild infection (white spots or a small, defined stain), apply topical over-the-counter antifungal agents to suppress the infection. Be aware, however, that these topical medications do not always penetrate the nail to reach the underlying infection. You'll need to take additional steps such as keeping the nail dry and allowing your feet to be exposed to the air as much as possible. If the stain does not disappear, and certainly if it spreads or starts to smell, seek medical attention. To diagnose your condition, your doctor may send tissue samples scraped from the nail to a laboratory in order to determine whether you have a fungal infection, and if so, how advanced it is. He or she may also remove the infected part of the nail through debridement (a gentle scraping of the nail surface). Depending on the extent of infection,

Table 1 Antifungal medications

GENERIC NAME	BRAND NAME(S)	HOW OFTEN TAKEN	POSSIBLE SIDE EFFECTS	COMMENTS
ciclopirox	Penlac Nail Lacquer	Applied directly to the nail and skin once a day	Rash; nail discoloration.	Topical treatment. Not as effective as oral medications, but has fewer side effects.
fluconazole	Diflucan	Taken orally once a day	Constipation; diarrhea; dizziness; drowsiness; headache; nausea, vomiting.	Interacts with many other medications, which may reduce effectiveness or increase side effects, so tell your doctor about all the medications you are taking.
griseofulvin	Fulvicin, Grifulvin, Gris-PEG	Taken orally twice a day	Headache; gastrointestinal problems; liver abnormalities after long-term use.	Available for more than 50 years; effective, but may require months of treatment.
itraconazole	Sporanox	Taken orally once or twice a day	Constipation; diarrhea; dizziness; drowsiness; headache; nausea, vomiting.	The FDA has warned that Sporanox may cause congestive heart failure and liver abnormalities. Your doctor may require regular liver and heart tests. Interacts with many other medications, which may reduce effectiveness or increase side effects, so tell your doctor about all the medications you are taking.
ketoconazole	Nizoral	Taken orally once a day	Constipation; diarrhea; dizziness; drowsiness; headache; nausea, vomiting.	Interacts with many other medications, which may reduce effectiveness or increase side effects, so tell your doctor about all the medications you are taking.
terbinafine	Lamisil	Taken orally once a day. Also available without prescription as a spray or cream for treatment of athlete's foot.	Diarrhea; nausea, vomiting; stomach pain; taste changes.	The FDA has warned that terbinafine may cause liver problems, although this is rare. To be safe, your doctor may require a baseline liver function test, followed by another test six to eight weeks after you begin treatment.

Note: Keep taking medication for the prescribed period, even if symptoms subside; fungal infections are tenacious.

your doctor may prescribe a topical or oral medication. For mild to moderate nail fungus, try a liquid form of ciclopirox (Penlac Nail Lacquer), which is the first topical medication specifically intended for fungal nails. This medication is applied daily, much like a nail polish, and complete treatment takes almost a year. During treatment, trim toenails yourself weekly and have a foot care professional trim them monthly.

Oral medications are also available (see Table 1), but the FDA has warned that two of these medications, itraconazole (Sporanox) and terbinafine (Lamisil), can cause serious liver damage and, in rare cases, death. Before giving you one of these medications, your doctor should do a baseline liver function test, as well as some other preliminary exams, to ensure that you are a candidate for an oral antifungal treatment. Your doctor may repeat the liver function test six to eight weeks after you start treatment. Sporanox has also been associated with a small risk of developing heart failure, and the FDA advises that it not be used at all by people who already have heart failure. All azole antifungal medications interact with many other drugs in ways that may reduce effectiveness or increase side effects, so mention all medications you are taking when you talk with your doctor about antifungal treatment. For example, taking itraconazole or ketoconazole (Nizoral) with one of the statin medications, such as atorvastatin (Lipitor) or simvastatin (Zocor), can cause serious muscular disorders.

Laser treatment is another method for treating fungal nail infections. To start, one or two laser applications are used to kill the fungus. But recurrence is common, and follow-up laser treatment may be needed.

If medications or laser treatments do not clear up your fungal infection, even after a second try, permanent surgical removal of the nail may be necessary. This will completely eradicate the infection, but your nail will not grow back afterward.

Athlete's foot

You don't have to be an athlete to develop athlete's foot, or tinea pedis, one of the most common types of fungal infection, affecting one in five adults. The condition, which affects men more often than women, is known

> **SYMPTOMS OF Athlete's foot**
> - White scales, especially around the toes
> - Itching and redness
> - Small rash-like blisters across the skin

as athlete's foot because walking around barefoot in a locker room is a good way to become infected. But you can also come in contact with the fungus in store dressing rooms, swimming pool changing areas, or any place that combines dampness and a lot of foot traffic. You can also be infected by improperly cleaned instruments used in a pedicure either at a commercial salon or at home (see "Pedicure precautions," page 31). Whatever the source, fungi thrive in dark, damp environments—for example, a sweaty foot in a shoe.

The types of fungi that cause athlete's foot are often the same ones that cause toenail fungus, although the infection manifests itself differently in the skin than in the nails. If you develop athlete's foot, you'll notice that the skin on your feet starts to develop white scaly patches or fissures, especially between the toes. As the infection progresses, the skin may turn red and become itchy. The skin will appear moist, not dry and scaly as in psoriasis. Small blisters may spread out across your foot, breaking to expose raw fissures that are painful and may swell. The area between the toes is most often affected, but the infection may spread to the soles of your feet or to your toenails, which can become thick and colored white or cloudy yellow. If you scratch your infected feet and then touch another part of your body, the infection may spread there as well. It can even contaminate bed sheets and reach parts of the body you're not aware of touching. In the most advanced cases, the rash will extend across the sole of your foot, and your feet may ooze pus and develop a foul odor.

The best way to prevent athlete's foot is by wearing sandals or shower shoes whenever you walk around a locker room or pool. Wash your feet with soap and water at least once a day, and keep your feet dry the rest of the time. Put on clean socks every day, and change them more often if you sweat a lot or get them wet. Give your feet a chance to "breathe": take your shoes off while at home, or wear sandals or canvas shoes that allow air to circulate. Avoid shoes or socks that make your feet sweat.

Treating athlete's foot

If you develop athlete's foot, you have numerous options. If the infection is mild (scaly white patches of skin or fissures, but no redness or itching), pay special attention to foot hygiene. Wash your feet regularly and dry them thoroughly, especially between the toes. Apply an antifungal cream to the affected area, and dust your socks and shoes with antifungal powder. Many effective remedies are available over the counter; look for products that contain clotrimazole, econazole, ketoconazole, miconazole, naftifine, oxiconazole, sulconazole, terbinafine, or terconazole. Brand names include Lamisil AT, Lotrimin, Micatin, and Tinactin. All are effective, but everyone differs in his or her response to particular ingredients, so if one doesn't work for you, try another. Follow the instructions that come with the medication.

Consult a foot care specialist if you see no improvement after two weeks of using over-the-counter remedies, if the infection is severe (the skin is red, itchy, peeling, or blistered), or if you have diabetes or some other circulatory problem. Your foot care specialist may prescribe a topical or oral medication to treat your athlete's foot. Even these will take several weeks to work. Athlete's foot can recur in some people, so even after it resolves, be sure to be vigilant about the preventive measures discussed above, and reapply medication at the first sign of recurrence. Oral medications, usually reserved for people with recurrent infections or infections that don't respond to topical treatment, include griseofulvin, itraconazole, and terbinafine. (For more information on these drugs, see Table 1.)

Warts

Anyone can get a wart. Warts result from infection with the human papillomavirus (HPV). When they appear on the soles of the feet, they are known as plantar warts, which are essentially the same as other warts except that, being compacted by the weight of the foot, they are hard and flat. Plantar warts may be gray or brown, with black spots in the center (although color varies widely). Warts on the top of the feet tend to be raised and spongy. Both types of warts may have a dimpled surface. For the most part, warts are not dangerous, but they can cause irritation and pain if exposed to pressure or friction, as is the case with many warts on the feet. Warts are also highly contagious, which means they are not only easy to catch but also easy to pass on. Children and teenagers are most likely to develop warts, but it's possible at any age.

To avoid warts, you have to avoid coming in contact with HPV (not to be confused with an entirely different strain of HPV that causes sexually transmitted diseases, such as genital warts and cervical cancer). You can protect yourself as much as possible by not walking barefoot on dirty surfaces, especially those that are moist and warm. Keep your feet clean and dry at all times. Change your socks every day. Do not touch or scratch a wart—either your own or someone else's—so as to avoid spreading it. Warm, moist towels provide perfect incubators for the virus, so use separate towels for drying your feet and the rest of your body, and don't share towels with someone who has a wart.

> ### ▶ SYMPTOMS OF Warts
>
> - Fleshy, raised, well-defined boundaries (on top of foot)
> - Hard, flat, well-defined boundaries (on bottom of foot)
> - Dimpled or rough surface
> - Varying color; may be gray or brown on bottom of foot, flesh-colored or pale on top of foot

Treating warts

If you notice a wart on your foot, one option is to do nothing. Sometimes warts disappear on their own—but some may not, depending on the size and depth of the wart. The risk of simply waiting for the wart to go away is that it may grow in size or seed other warts across the foot. Most people prefer to do something, especially if shoes or the pressure of walking cause the wart to itch or hurt.

Unless you have diabetes or some other underlying medical condition that makes you prone to infections or slow to heal, your next option is an over-the-counter preparation that includes 40% salicylic acid (Clear Away, Compound W, others). Follow the directions carefully. These products contain acids or chemicals that destroy skin, and you risk damaging healthy skin along with the wart. Using these products can be a long, laborious process. You may need to apply the medication every day for weeks or months, scraping off the dead skin the following day. Another option is to consult a foot care specialist, who may apply a stronger topical preparation.

A quicker but more painful option is to have your doctor remove the wart by freezing it, a procedure known as cryotherapy. The frozen tissue then dies and falls off, like a scab. No anesthetic is used in cryotherapy. There will be no pain while the wart is actually frozen, but you may feel some pain for a short time as it thaws. Sometimes, you may have to go a second time, if the entire wart wasn't removed or if it grows back. Your doctor may also perform outpatient surgery, excising the wart with a scalpel under local anesthetic. Another procedure uses a carbon dioxide laser to remove the wart, again with a local anesthetic.

A less painful option is pulse-dye laser removal. This technique may not be available everywhere, but it is worth asking your doctor about. The pulse-dye laser emits a beam of light that targets and destroys red blood cells in the wart. This deprives the wart of access to oxygen and nutrients but does not harm the surrounding skin and tissue. It usually takes three treatments with the laser, three weeks apart, to destroy the wart completely. Before each laser treatment, the thick skin of the wart is shaved (debrided) to better

▶ Pedicure precautions

A pedicure is a great way to pamper your feet, but be aware that state regulations and licensing requirements for professional salons vary and are not always well enforced. If you go to a salon, make sure the pedicurist sterilizes any instruments thoroughly to reduce the chance of passing on a toenail fungus. Reusable instruments should be disinfected for at least 10 minutes in either an FDA-approved high-level disinfectant solution or in a disinfectant registered with the Environmental Protection Agency, then stored in a clean, dry container. The safest option is for the salon to use disposable instruments, which are discarded after each client. Many doctors recommend that you bring your own instruments to a commercial pedicurist. Devices like whirlpool foot baths that are shared by clients also need to be disinfected regularly. Finally, to avoid getting an infection, do not let a pedicurist file corns or calluses or use any sharp instrument on your feet.

If you'd rather try a pedicure at home (or if you wish to purchase your own tools), you can usually find a basic kit at your local pharmacy. It should include orange sticks, foam separators for toes, files, and emery boards, as well as lotions, soaps, and soaks. You can use a pumice stone or a file to gently remove calluses. These directions may help:

- **Fill a pan or basin with warm water.** You can also add Epsom salts, oils, or mild cleansers.
- **Soak your feet for five minutes or so,** until the skin and nails soften.
- **Dry your feet with a towel.** Don't forget your toes and the areas between them.
- **Gently rub a pumice stone against your skin,** paying special attention to your heels and toes, to remove any dead skin cells. Be careful not to rub too hard, or you'll damage the skin.

- **Take care of the cuticles.** First, rub lotion or oil onto your toenails to soften the cuticles (the thin layer of skin at the bottom and sides of your toenail). Then gently push the cuticles back to the base of the nails, using an orange stick or a moist washcloth. Don't cut the cuticles; that could lead to infection.
- **Clean underneath your nails** with an orange stick wrapped in cotton or soaked in water to soften the edge. (Try not to use metal sticks or nail files, which might cut your skin and lead to infection.)
- **Cut your toenails straight across** with a toe clipper, or by making a series of small snips with nail scissors. Smooth the edges of any rough nails with an emery board.
- **Apply foot lotion to your feet,** rubbing it gently into the skin. If you are going to apply nail polish, wipe excess lotion from the toenails using a cotton ball soaked with rubbing alcohol.
- **Apply nail polish.** First, use foam toe separators or cotton balls to separate your toes. Then apply the polish. Allow each coat to dry for several minutes. Wait an hour before putting on socks and shoes, so the nail polish won't smudge or chip.
- **Clean up.** If you share your pedicure kit with someone else, throw away the emery board and orange stick. (If you're the only person using the kit, you can keep them in a clean, dry place.) Scrub any metal tools, such as toe clippers or scissors, with soap and water; then disinfect them in an antibacterial solution. Again, if you are the only person who uses them, cleaning and disinfecting with alcohol, Lysol, or peroxide should be sufficient. Clean the basin in the same manner.

expose blood vessels to the laser. Each pulse of the laser causes a brief, sharp pain, similar to an elastic band hitting the skin, and a mild burning sensation afterward. A local anesthetic can be used to numb the area ahead of time if you don't think you can tolerate the discomfort. Although the pulse-dye laser is considered an effective noninvasive method of wart removal, it is not for everyone. The technique works best on warts that have red dots, are scaly in texture, and have not been previously treated.

Yet another option to consider is topical fluorouracil (Carac, Efudex, Fluoroplex), a prescription cream originally developed to treat certain kinds of skin cancer. Because this medication works on skin conditions in which cells are multiplying rapidly, it has also been used to treat psoriasis, genital warts, and warts on the feet. One pilot study, conducted in children, found it to be effective in eliminating warts; other investigators aren't convinced. But if you prefer medication to surgery, ask your doctor about it.

Other health conditions

Although most of the foot conditions described in this report are easily treated, some can become serious and threaten your quality of life if you suffer from diabetes, nerve damage, or a vascular problem that interferes with the healing of injuries. And anyone can get skin cancer, which can originate as a spot anywhere on the foot—including the sole—but is often overlooked until it spreads.

Diabetes

If you have diabetes, be particularly careful about foot health. The prolonged effects of diabetes and elevated blood sugar may eventually damage not only vital organs like the heart and kidneys, but also nerves and blood vessels, including those that serve the feet. The nerve damage caused by diabetes can lead to peripheral neuropathy, which may make your feet less sensitive to irritation and pain. As a result, you may not be aware of the discomfort of ill-fitting shoes, or you may not realize that you have suffered a foot injury, allowing the situation to worsen. Diabetes can also impair your circulation, impeding your natural healing capacity and your ability to fight infection.

By some estimates, as many as 15% of people with diabetes will develop a foot ulcer at some point in their lives, and 6% of those who do will be hospitalized because of a related complication, such as an infection. All too often, the problem worsens to the point where a toe, a foot, or even a leg will need to be amputated. More than 60% of lower leg amputations occur in people with diabetes, yet the Centers for Disease Control and Prevention estimates that as many as 85% of these amputations could be avoided if people with diabetes took care of their feet and had regular foot examinations. Public awareness aimed at educating those with diabetes about prevention may be making an impact. Since 1996, the number of people ages 40 or older with diabetes who were hospitalized for foot amputation declined by 65%, according to a 2012 study published in *Diabetes Care*. The reason for the decline is probably a combination of improved blood sugar control, better foot care, and a lower prevalence of cardiovascular disease. See a doctor immediately if you notice any warning signs (see "Symptoms of diabetes-associated foot problems," below).

Caring for your feet

Recognizing the devastating impact of diabetic foot problems, the American College of Foot and Ankle Surgeons in 2006 updated its guidelines for caring for people with diabetes to place greater emphasis on prevention. Although these guidelines were written for physicians, we have adapted them here for use by patients with diabetes who want to protect their feet.

- **Know your feet.** Take a good look every day to see if you've cut or bruised your feet without realizing it. Pay attention to any growths or discoloration. If your foot swells or changes in color, for example, it could be a sign of a fractured bone or poor circulation.

- **Practice good foot hygiene.** Wash your feet every day. Dry them thoroughly, especially between the toes. Moisturize any dry skin (but not between your toes), or dust with foot powder to keep your feet dry. Cut the nails straight across to avoid ingrown toenails, which can lead to infection. However, be careful when wielding the scissors: if you've lost sensation in your feet, or if your nails have grown harder, consider having your nails trimmed professionally.

> ▶ **SYMPTOMS OF Diabetes-associated foot problems**
>
> - Changes in the color of your feet
> - Swelling or pain in your feet or legs
> - Cracks in the skin, especially around your heels
> - Open sores anywhere on your feet
> - Wounds that don't heal

- **Protect your feet.** Wear shoes with ample cushioning and socks that protect against friction. Make sure your shoes fit by having your foot measured every time you buy a new pair (see "What to look for in a shoe," page 45). Shoes cause a large number of all diabetic complications that lead to amputation. Avoid high heels or shoes with pointy toes. If you must wear such shoes for dressy occasions, try to limit the amount of time they are on your feet.

- **Practice overall good health.** If you need to, try to lose weight. Every extra pound increases the pressure on your feet. Don't smoke—smoking impairs circulation. Exercise regularly to improve circulation.

- **Drink in moderation.** Avoid excessive consumption of alcohol, which can impair nerves already at risk because of diabetes. Government health agencies and the American Medical Association define moderate drinking as no more than two standard drinks per day for men under age 65 and one drink per day for women, as well as for men 65 and older. (A drink is defined as 12 ounces of beer, 5 ounces of wine, or 1.5 ounces of hard liquor.)

- **Learn when to seek help.** If you have diabetes, you're also more prone to complications. If you develop any of the foot problems described in this report, it's vital that you see a doctor. Don't try to treat yourself at home—you may end up making the problem worse. To prevent problems from developing, see a foot care specialist at least once a year to have your feet evaluated.

- **Apply for Medicare-funded shoes.** Medicare covers the cost of therapeutic shoes and inserts for people with diabetes, in an effort to reduce foot and leg amputations. Medicare covers 80% of the approved cost of the shoes, after you have met the $100 annual deductible for durable equipment (which can also include insulin pumps and other therapeutic devices). If you qualify, you are eligible for molded shoes, which are custom-designed to fit your foot snugly, or depth shoes, which provide extra support to the arch. Inserts are included with both types of shoes. Ask your doctor about the Medicare program, because the shoes must be ordered through a physician or podiatrist. Or call the Medicare Helpline at 800-633-4227 (toll-free) for more information.

Figure 6 A view of Morton's neuroma

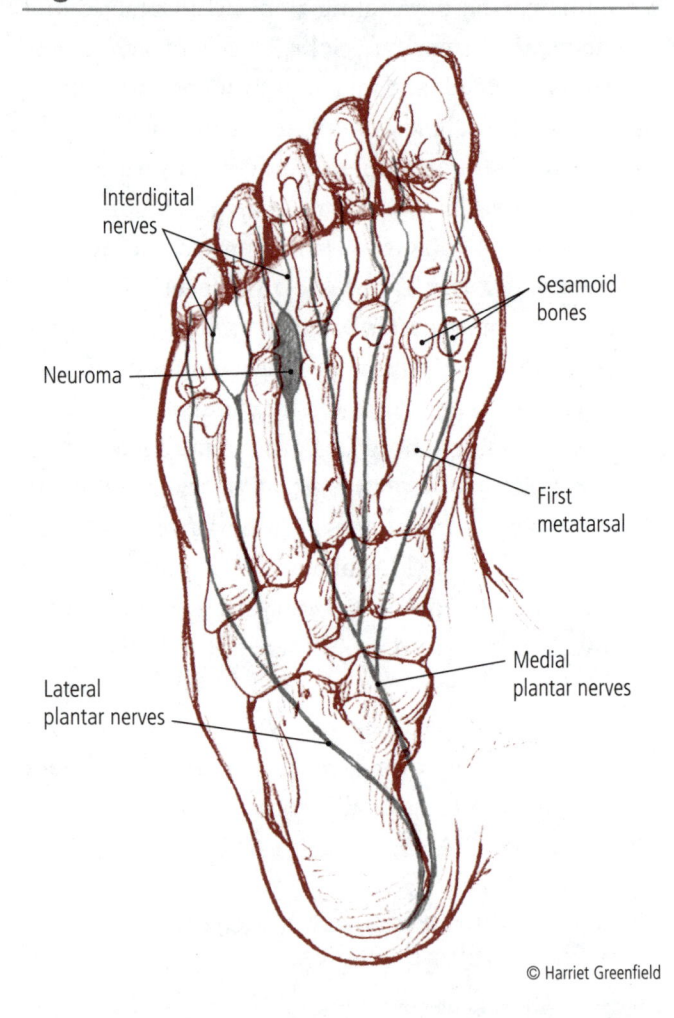

© Harriet Greenfield

Along the bottom of the foot, the nerves of the toes pass between the metatarsal bones. As a result of tight-fitting shoes or activities such as jogging or dancing, these nerves can be compressed by the bones and become irritated. The area between the third and fourth toes is the most common site for this condition, which is named Morton's neuroma after the doctor who first described it.

Nerve problems

Two types of nerve problems most commonly affect the foot: a neuroma, also known as a pinched or swollen nerve, and peripheral neuropathy, which involves more widespread damage to nerves due to a systemic condition such as diabetes.

Morton's neuroma

A neuroma develops when a nerve is compressed, injured, or pinched, causing swelling and pain. The nerves most often affected in the feet are branches of the plantar nerves, which supply feeling to the bottoms of the feet and toes. A neuroma in the area between the third and fourth toes or between the second and third toes is particularly common and is known as a Morton's neuroma (see Figure 6). Women are roughly seven times more likely to develop a Morton's neuroma than men. At greatest risk are women ages 30 to 60 who wear tight shoes.

Morton's neuroma causes a combination of sharp, burning pain (often described as shooting or electric, like intense pins and needles) and numbness in the toes and foot. Typically it flares up when you are standing. You may feel like you've stepped on a tiny hot coal and can't get rid of it, while at the same time having the disconcerting experience of not being able to feel your toes. Sometimes the nerve tissue becomes so thickened you can feel or see a lump.

To prevent Morton's neuroma, wear shoes with wide toe boxes. Tight, pointy shoes are the principal culprits behind neuromas. These shoes squeeze bones, ligaments, muscles, and nerves. High heels may aggravate the problem by shifting your weight forward. Over time, this combination can cause the nerves to swell and become painful. There are other, less frequent causes of Morton's neuroma: injury to the foot, repeated trauma (seen among professional ballet dancers), or certain inborn structural defects that place too much pressure on the nerves of the foot.

■ **Treating Morton's neuroma.** The first step in treating a neuroma is to wear shoes that provide enough room in the toe box. For instant relief when pain flares up, some people find it useful to take their shoes off and rub the area; this can provide relief because the nerve can get trapped below the ligament, and the manipulation can move it back to its natural position. Your foot care specialist may recommend lower heels, metatarsal pads, and better arch support to redistribute your weight. Custom orthoses will help correct structural problems and will distribute the pressure more evenly. If you're in severe pain, your doctor may give you an injection of a local anesthetic combined with a corticosteroid to relieve the inflammation and pain. If you keep pressure off the toes and wear wide enough shoes, the problem may gradually disappear.

For severe or persistent pain, you may require surgery to remove the neuroma. Traditionally this has involved making an incision in the foot and performing open neurectomy, or removal of the nerve. A less invasive type of surgery, called endoscopic decompression, involves a smaller incision and may hasten your recovery time. Be aware that once the nerve is gone, you permanently lose feeling in the affected area.

It's also important to realize that, with any type of neuroma surgery, complications may occur. First of all, part of the nerve remains after surgery. In a small percentage of people, pain develops in the remaining "nub" of normal nerve tissue, a problem known as stump neuroma. Another possible and very rare complication is the development of complex regional pain syndrome, characterized by severe pain in the foot that was operated on, sometimes spreading to the entire leg. Researchers aren't sure why this develops after nerve surgery, but when it does occur, it usually results in lifelong pain that must be managed with medications.

One alternative to surgery, if you continue to have pain from a neuroma, is to undergo neurolysis injections, which use various chemical agents to block pain signals. Although some foot care specialists offer this therapy, evidence about its effectiveness is limited. Another alternative to surgery is to take a prescription pain reliever that alleviates nerve pain, such as amitriptyline (Elavil), gabapentin (Neurontin), or pregabalin (Lyrica). More information about these medications appears in Table 2 (see page 41).

Peripheral neuropathy

The nervous system has two parts. The central nervous system consists of the brain and spinal cord, while the peripheral nervous system consists of the nerves that fan out to the rest of the body and relay sensory information to and from the skin, organs, and extremities—including the feet. Peripheral neuropathy occurs when nerves in the peripheral system suffer damage or degenerate. The condition can develop for any number of reasons. Diabetes is a leading culprit. About 60% to 70% of Americans with diabetes experience peripheral neuropathy, according to the 2011 Centers for Disease Control and Prevention National Diabetes Fact Sheet.

Other causes include excessive alcohol consumption over a prolonged period, dietary deficiencies (caused by poor absorption of B vitamins), physical trauma, prolonged compression, vascular problems such as atherosclerosis (hardening of the arteries), and immune system disorders like rheumatoid arthritis or systemic lupus erythematosus.

The symptoms of peripheral neuropathy are as diverse as the causes. The condition can cause a burning, shooting pain through your hands or feet. Sometimes the pain will wake you up at night, or it may feel more intense when you are resting. Another version, motor neuropathy, affects the nerves that instruct your muscles to move. It can cause weakness in your leg and foot muscles, which can lead to structural deformities such as bunions or hammertoes. Other symptoms include tingling and numbness in the feet, or even tickling or other abnormal sensations.

To determine the severity of your peripheral nerve damage, your doctor may do a nerve conduction test, which involves placing electrodes on your feet to see whether nerve signals are being transmitted in a normal pattern. This involves a very low level of electricity and should not hurt.

■ **Treating peripheral neuropathy.** If you have peripheral neuropathy, regardless of the cause, it's important to pay extra attention to your feet. Examine them at least once a day to be sure that you haven't developed a sore or lesion. Since your nerves may no longer communicate pain efficiently, you need to rely on your eyes to detect any problems.

Because there are many causes of peripheral neuropathy, treatment varies according to the primary problem. If the cause is diabetes, treatment aims at better control of high blood sugar levels, which can damage blood vessels that nourish the nerves and interfere with a nerve's ability to transmit signals. If the problem is compression by a tumor or some underlying structural problem, surgery may be in order. Vitamin deficiency is corrected with regular injections of B vitamins.

Your recovery will depend on the amount of damage that occurred before the problem was corrected. In very rare cases, the nerve will return to normal slowly, and you won't have any lasting effects. Most of the time, however, lingering sensory or motor abnormalities will remain, and the goal of treatment will be to prevent further damage. Nerve pain medications, such as duloxetine (Cymbalta)—an antidepressant medication approved by the FDA in 2004 to manage nerve pain associated with diabetes—may also offer some relief, as may pregabalin (Lyrica), a neuropathic pain reliever (see Table 2). Metanx, a prescription medication used to treat diabetic neuropathy, may also help. Metanx contains active forms of folate, vitamin B_6, and B_{12}. According to its manufacturer, Metanx works by increasing the body's natural production of nitric acid, which in turn helps dilate blood vessels, increasing blood flow to the peripheral vessels and nerves.

Skin cancer

The last place you might think to check for a suspicious mole is the sole of your foot, but most people don't realize that even the underside of the foot gets exposed to the sun and is vulnerable to melanoma and other types of skin cancer. The incidence of melanoma is increasing. Melanoma can occur anywhere on the foot—even in between toes and underneath toenails. Melanoma was responsible for 76,250 new cases of skin cancer and 9,180 deaths in 2011, and it is increasing at a faster rate than any other cancer in the United States, particularly in young women ages 15 to 39.

Since melanoma of the foot is usually noticed late by patients, and more likely to be misdiagnosed by doctors than melanoma in any other location, it typically isn't recognized and treated until it has advanced or metastasized to other parts of the body, which makes prognosis for survival poor. Studies have consistently linked melanoma of the foot with a lower than average survival rate. (The survival rate for melanoma anywhere else on the body is 80% to 85%.) One study that looked at survival followed 148 patients with melanoma originating on a lower extremity. The malignant lesion was located on the foot or ankle in 37 participants, and on the leg, knee, or thigh of 111 patients. The overall survival rate was 52% for patients with a primary melanoma of the foot or ankle, compared with 84% for patients with a melanoma located elsewhere on the leg. According to the American College of Foot and Ankle Surgeons (ACFAS), half of all people diagnosed with melanoma of the foot will die within five years because of late diagnosis.

Inspect your feet

Early detection is essential to successful treatment of melanoma, so take the time to regularly examine your feet—including the tops, soles, under toenails, and in between toes. The ACFAS recommends doing so every time you trim your toenails. When checking out your feet, look for any mole, freckle, or spot that may have changed over the course of the month or meets the guidelines for identifying melanoma (see "The ABCDEs of melanoma," at right). If you wear nail polish consistently, be sure to take it off periodically so you can see underneath the nail, where discoloration of any size or shape is cause for concern—especially if you've noticed it hasn't grown out with the nail. Melanomas on the feet are commonly mistaken for—and even misdiagnosed as—nail fungus, ulcers, or hematomas. Recognizing them may not be easy, so talk with a foot specialist or dermatologist about any spot that concerns you.

Protect your feet

It's easy to forget your feet when you put on sunscreen, but if you're wearing sandals or going barefoot, be sure to apply sunscreen to the tops and soles of the feet as well as in between your toes. Wearing water shoes in the summer that cover your feet, rather than flip-flops or sandals that expose them, is helpful. So is avoiding sun exposure during the peak hours of 10 a.m. and 2 p.m., when ultraviolet rays are strongest.

Vascular problems and cold feet

Vascular conditions affect the arteries that carry blood throughout your body. Many people suffer poor circulation, especially as they grow older, and this may lead to cold feet. High blood pressure (hypertension) and other types of cardiovascular disease can also reduce circulation, especially to the extremities. So can phlebitis, an inflammation of a vein that sometimes causes a blood clot.

Treating vascular problems and cold feet

If you notice that your feet are colder than usual, visit your doctor to determine whether it's a sign of a heart or circulatory problem. Treatment of any underlying condition, be it phlebitis or high blood pressure, may help restore circulation and is important for your overall health. You can also help yourself by getting more exercise, because activity improves circulation. It may help to massage your feet regularly, either with your hands or by rolling your feet over nubby objects (see "Foot massage," page 40), which helps draw blood into the area.

The ABCDEs of melanoma

If a spot on your foot meets any of the criteria below, be sure to see a foot specialist or dermatologist right away.

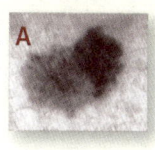

Asymmetry. Most moles have a round, symmetrical shape, but melanoma is asymmetrical, meaning one side may be different in shape than the other.

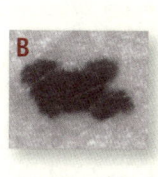

Border irregularity. Normal moles are round and typically have a clear border. In melanoma, the borders are shabby, uneven, or indistinct, sometimes blending into the surrounding skin. A mole resembling the shape of cauliflower, for instance, should be checked out.

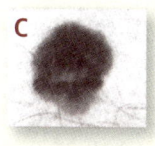

Color. Melanomas are usually very dark, but often are a mix of hues rather than one color.

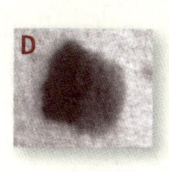

Diameter. Most common moles are small, less than 5 millimeters, which is about a quarter of an inch. Melanoma grows, so talk to your doctor if the spot is larger than the one pictured here.

Evolving. Look for any change in size, shape, color, or elevation, or any new symptoms such as bleeding, itching, or crusting.

Foot surgery

Because the foot has so many bones, joints, muscles, tendons, ligaments, and blood vessels, foot surgery can be lengthy, and recovery may take longer than you'd expect. As with any operation, foot surgery involves risks such as infection, nerve injury, postoperative pain, scar formation, and complications from anesthesia. Even so, there are times when foot surgery is your best option. Modern advances in surgical techniques and equipment have significantly improved outcomes for patients. But don't book that tennis match right away. Although your problem might be fixed, remember that full recovery from any surgical procedure on the foot takes time. Most healing occurs within the first several weeks after surgery, but it may take as long as three to six months, and sometimes more, depending on the procedure, before the injured area is strong enough to take on high-impact activities.

Types of surgical procedures

The following surgical techniques are frequently used in foot surgery.

■ **Arthroscopy/endoscopy.** Minimally invasive surgery may shorten a patient's recovery time and often can be done on an outpatient basis. In a procedure called arthroscopy, the surgeon makes a tiny incision and inserts an arthroscope, a pen-sized instrument with a miniature video camera on the end. This device sends images to a monitor, enabling the surgeon to see inside your joint while operating with very small surgical tools. Endoscopy is a closely related procedure that uses a lighted scope called an endoscope to show the inside of a body cavity. In foot surgery, it is most often used for an operation to release the plantar fascia in treating plantar fasciitis, although it may also be used to treat Morton's neuroma.

■ **Bone fusion (arthrodesis).** In this procedure, your surgeon removes the cartilage of a joint and uses pins, screws, or plates to rigidly bind together the two bones that made up the joint. As the bones heal, they grow together as one bone. Arthrodesis is quite effective at reducing the pain of arthritis, but you won't be able to move the joint afterward. The procedure can be used anywhere in the foot.

■ **Bony reconstruction.** With reconstructive procedures, the bones of the foot are realigned, often by making cuts in the bone. After they are repositioned, the bones are usually held in place with plates, screws, or both. Examples of such reconstructive procedures include the correction of bunions and rigid flat foot deformities.

■ **Soft tissue repair.** As your feet age, your muscles, tendons, and ligaments may weaken or degrade, providing less support to the bones. This can lead to painful deformities. Your surgeon may repair the damage by tightening, loosening, or realigning the imbalanced tissues. Examples of such procedures include the correction of flexible toe or flat foot deformities.

■ **Arthroplasty (joint replacement).** With this procedure, implants are used to replace joints damaged by arthritis in the ankle or at the joint of the big toe. Although performed routinely on the hip or knee, joint replacement in the foot is a technique that is still evolving.

Having foot surgery

Today, some surgical procedures on the foot are performed on an outpatient basis, which means you'll be released the day of the surgery. Many procedures can be performed in a doctor's office, rather than in a hospital. Generally, anesthesia for foot surgery is either local (affecting only part of the foot) or regional (numbing the entire foot). The method chosen depends on your particular foot problem, the procedure, your overall medical condition, and your preferences. Discuss the options with your foot surgeon. After the operation, you'll be given pain medication to use at home while you recover—often a prescription medication, such as one containing codeine (see Table 2, page 41).

After the operation, the area will be covered with a bandage. Depending on the procedure, you may have to wear a special surgical shoe or a plaster cast to protect your foot while it heals. You may also be sent to a physical therapist to help you regain function and mobility in the foot. Your doctor may prescribe home exercises to strengthen your foot and keep it flexible.

Cosmetic foot surgery

Cosmetic procedures include operations that shorten perfectly normal toes or correct other real or perceived flaws in appearance, often for the express purpose of fitting into fashionable high-heeled shoes. Although such procedures may improve the outer appearance of the foot, they do nothing to lessen pain or improve your ability to walk—the usual reasons for undergoing surgery. In fact, complications from surgery can lead to chronic foot pain. In a survey of orthopedic surgeons—all members of the American Orthopaedic Foot and Ankle Society (AOFAS)—50% said they've treated patients for foot problems caused by complications from cosmetic foot surgery.

Although some media articles and advertisements make it seem as though cosmetic foot surgery is no big deal, it's wise to think carefully before agreeing to such a procedure. Cosmetic foot surgery can be expensive, yet insurance plans typically do not cover these procedures, so patients must pay out of pocket. What's more, both the AOFAS and the American Podiatric Medical Association have strongly advised against undergoing cosmetic foot surgery. Any surgery, no matter how minor, is associated with risks that can range from infection to impairment. The two main goals and benefits of foot surgery are to relieve pain and improve function. Cosmetic foot surgery does neither and is therefore considered medically unwarranted, given the potentially serious risks involved.

Treating foot pain

Pain is a symptom common to many foot conditions. Pain medications are a good solution for most types of foot pain. You also can try other approaches, either before resorting to pain relievers or in conjunction with them. For example, you can try an ice pack or a warm foot soak before reaching for the pain pills. In general, if your skin feels warm to the touch (indicating that your foot is inflamed), apply ice (see "First aid: The RICE regimen," page 22). Don't apply warmth to an inflamed area because it will only increase the blood flow and make the inflammation worse.

If your feet are tired and sore and your skin feels normal or cool to the touch, try soaking your feet in a warm bath to relax and soothe them. Pharmacies sell gel packs that you can either freeze or heat in the microwave, then apply to your feet. You can also try foot massage (see page box, left). Gently rubbing sore muscles and joints can often provide needed relief. But don't massage a foot that is inflamed or that you think might be injured.

When it comes to pharmaceutical treatment, there are a number of different options. Some medications are topical—that is, you apply them to the skin. Others are systemic; these are usually taken in pill form. A summary of the major categories of pain relief medications follows. (For more information on specific drugs, see Table 2.)

■ **Analgesics.** This class of medications encompasses pain relievers such as acetaminophen (Tylenol), which relieve pain without relieving inflammation. Be aware that doctors caution people who drink heavily against using acetaminophen because alcohol can combine with this drug to cause liver damage.

■ **Topical analgesics.** Topical pain medications are available in lotion, cream, or gel form. They are spread on the skin and penetrate inward to relieve some forms of mild foot pain. Some topical preparations—such as those containing menthol, eucalyptus oil, or turpentine oil—reduce pain by distracting the nerves with a different type of sensation. Another group delivers salicylates (the same ingredient as in aspirin) through the skin. A third group contains a chemical known as substance P, which is a neurotransmitter that appears to transmit pain signals to the brain. These creams contain a derivative of a natural ingredient found in cayenne pepper. For that reason, they may burn or sting when first applied.

■ **Nonsteroidal anti-inflammatory drugs (NSAIDs).** NSAIDs are available both with and without a prescription. Popular over-the-counter NSAIDs include aspirin (Bayer, Bufferin, others), ibuprofen (Advil, Motrin, oth-

Foot massage

Your feet may benefit from a regular rubdown. Some people massage their own feet; others ask someone for help. Massage improves circulation, stimulates muscles, reduces tension, and may alleviate pain. Don't massage your feet if you have an injury or any sign of infection or inflammation, such as redness or swelling. When you massage your feet, take the time to examine them, and report any sign of problems to your doctor. Here's how to do a massage:

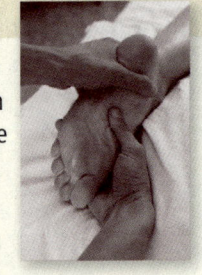

- Sit in a comfortable chair. Bend your left leg and rest your left foot gently on your right thigh.
- Pour some skin lotion or oil into your hand. Rub it gently into your foot and massage your whole foot—toes, arch, and heel.
- Do a deeper massage. Press the knuckles of your right hand into your left foot. Knead your foot as you would bread. Or work the skin and muscles by holding a foot with both hands and pressing your thumbs into the skin.
- Using your hands, gently pull the toes back and forth or apart. This stretches the muscles underneath.
- Repeat on the other foot.

To enhance your massage, you can buy massage devices in local drugstores or health stores. Foot rollers can provide fast foot massages at home or at work—take off your shoes and roll your feet over the massagers for a quick pick-me-up.

Table 2 Medications for foot pain

GENERIC NAME	BRAND NAME(S)	HOW OFTEN TAKEN	POSSIBLE SIDE EFFECTS	COMMENTS
Over-the-counter medications				
acetaminophen	Tylenol, others	4–6 hours	When taken as directed, does not usually cause side effects. In excessively high doses, may damage the liver.	Useful for mild pain. Not an NSAID; does not reduce inflammation. Heavy drinkers should consult a doctor about possible interactions.
aspirin (acetylsalicylic acid)	Bayer, Bufferin, others	4–6 hours	Abdominal pain, gastric ulcers, heartburn, indigestion, nausea, vomiting, ringing in ears.	An NSAID.* Interferes with blood clotting; do not use with blood thinners or before surgery.
ibuprofen	Advil, Motrin IB, others	4–6 hours	Gastrointestinal effects similar to but less pronounced than those associated with aspirin. Discuss your personal health with your doctor when considering regular use.	An NSAID.* Do not take for more than 10 days for pain or more than three days for fever unless your doctor tells you to.
naproxen	Aleve	8–12 hours	Gastrointestinal effects similar to those of aspirin or ibuprofen. Discuss use of this drug with your doctor.	An NSAID.* Derived from propionic acid, like ibuprofen, but stays in the bloodstream longer. Do not take for more than 10 days for pain or more than three days for fever unless your doctor tells you to.
Prescription NSAIDs*				
diclofenac	Cataflam / Voltaren	6–12 hours / 6–8 hours	Abdominal pain, gastric ulcers, bleeding, drowsiness, dizziness, fluid retention, heartburn, indigestion, rash, ringing in ears, kidney damage, liver damage. Discuss use of these drugs with your doctor.	Long-term use can cause gastrointestinal side effects.*
ibuprofen	Motrin	6–8 hours		
naproxen	Naprosyn	12 hours		

*All NSAIDs should be taken with a glass of milk, food, or an antacid to reduce the likelihood of gastrointestinal distress. If you cannot take aspirin or suffer from asthma, high blood pressure, peptic ulcers, or kidney or liver disorders, check with your doctor before taking an NSAID. Do not take NSAIDs if you are taking blood thinners. If you drink more than three alcoholic beverages a day, do not use NSAIDs before checking with your doctor.

GENERIC NAME	BRAND NAME(S)	HOW OFTEN TAKEN	POSSIBLE SIDE EFFECTS	COMMENTS
COX-2 inhibitor				
celecoxib	Celebrex	12–24 hours	Abdominal pain, drowsiness, dizziness, fluid retention, heartburn, indigestion, rash, ringing in ears, kidney damage, liver damage, cardiovascular effects. Discuss your personal health risks with your doctor when considering regular use.	Offers pain relief similar to prescription NSAIDs. Do not take in combination with NSAIDs. If you have high blood pressure or heart disease, talk with your doctor before taking.
Opioid analgesics (most often prescribed for postoperative pain following foot surgery)				
acetaminophen with codeine	Tylenol with codeine, others	4 hours	Constipation, dizziness, nausea or vomiting, sleepiness.	Take with food or milk. Do not drive an automobile or operate heavy machinery while taking this medication. May lead to physical or emotional dependence. Do not use if you have a history of substance abuse.
oxycodone	OxyContin (sustained release), Percocet, Roxicet, Roxicodone	3–8 hours, depending on drug and dose	Dizziness, drowsiness, nausea or vomiting, unusual tiredness, stomach pain.	Do not use if you are currently taking antidepressants, antihistamines, or other medications that affect the central nervous system. Do not use if you have a history of substance abuse. Do not drive or operate heavy machinery.
tramadol (non-narcotic)	Ultram	6 hours	Constipation, dizziness, headache, nausea, sleepiness.	Do not use if you have a history of substance abuse or if you suffer from asthma, kidney problems, or liver problems.

Table 2 Medications for foot pain (continued)

Medications for nerve pain

GENERIC NAME	BRAND NAME(S)	HOW OFTEN TAKEN	POSSIBLE SIDE EFFECTS	COMMENTS
amitriptyline	Elavil	10–26 hours	Dizziness, drowsiness, dry mouth, headache, nausea, weight gain.	Amitriptyline is an antidepressant, but can also relieve nerve pain; it blocks nerve pathways that are involved in both depression and pain.
gabapentin	Neurontin	5–7 hours	Clumsiness, continuous eye movements, mood changes.	Follow doctor's instructions exactly. Medication dose increases gradually over first three days, then is maintained at a therapeutic level.
pregabalin	Lyrica	6 hours	Dizziness, dry mouth, drowsiness, headache, weight gain.	Limits pain from damaged nerves; also used to control seizures in epilepsy. Do not take while drinking alcohol, as this may increase side effects.
L-methylfolate, vitamin B_6, vitamin B_{12}	Metanx	Once or twice daily	Nausea, stomach upset, diarrhea, drowsiness, and numbness/tingling.	Helps maintain blood flow to blood vessels that carry vital nutrients and oxygen to the nerves of the foot.
duloxetine	Cymbalta	Once a day	Nausea, dry mouth, constipation, loss of appetite, tiredness, drowsiness, dizziness, increased sweating, blurred vision, or yawning.	A serotonin-norepinephrine reuptake inhibitor (SNRI), prescribed primarily as an antidepressant, that works by helping to restore the balance of certain substances in the brain (neurotransmitters). May improve mood, sleep, appetite, and energy level, and decrease nervousness. Can also decrease pain caused by nerve damage.

ers), and naproxen (Aleve, others). If you are taking an NSAID solely to relieve pain, expect to take a low dosage for a limited amount of time—usually until the pain is gone. If you have a condition that involves inflammation as well as pain, such as Achilles' tendinitis or a sprain, your doctor may advise you to take an NSAID at a higher dose and for a longer period, sometimes as much as several weeks. Why the difference? You can feel the pain-relieving effects of NSAIDs almost immediately, but you do not experience the full anti-inflammatory effects until a sufficient amount of the medication builds up in your bloodstream. Be aware that NSAID medications have a variety of side effects, so it is important to discuss your personal health risks with your doctor when considering their regular use.

■ **COX-2 inhibitor.** A type of prescription NSAID known as a COX-2 inhibitor, such as celecoxib (Celebrex), relieves pain and inflammation and may reduce the risk for gastric ulcers and bleeding, which sometimes make older NSAIDs difficult to tolerate. COX-2 inhibitors have their own side effects, though, so discuss your personal health risks with your doctor when considering the long-term use of these medications.

■ **Opioid analgesics.** Prescription drugs that contain opioids such as codeine are useful for pain that can't be relieved by analgesics or NSAIDs. They provide stronger pain relief because they block certain chemical pathways that send pain signals through the central nervous system. Many of these medications also cause drowsiness.

■ **Nerve pain medications.** Pain caused by nerve damage may not respond well to the usual pain relievers, so doctors rely on other medications. Two mainstays in treating nerve pain in the feet include the antidepressant amitriptyline (Elavil), which increases the levels of brain chemicals that ratchet down pain signals, and the anticonvulsant gabapentin (Neurontin), which apparently works by interfering with nerve signaling involved in pain as well as seizures. In 2004, the FDA approved pregabalin (Lyrica), a medication for nerve pain relief that also doubles as an antiseizure medication, and duloxetine (Cymbalta), an antidepressant, for nerve pain associated with diabetes.

■ **Nerve blocks.** A nerve block is an injection that numbs a particular nerve to prevent pain signals from reaching your brain (much as lidocaine does in a dentist's office). It's effective for severe pain or for use during a surgical procedure.

■ **Corticosteroids.** These medications are synthetic forms of naturally occurring hormones produced by the adrenal glands. Corticosteroids may be given in the form of pills or injections to decrease inflammation and thus relieve pain. Topical corticosteroids, applied directly to the skin, are useful only in treating rashes, not for pain due to musculoskeletal injuries.

■ **Ultrasound.** This is not a medication, but rather a treatment in which high-frequency sound waves are directed at an inflamed area to speed healing and reduce inflammation. It works best on soft-tissue injuries. ▼

Shoes for healthy feet

If there's a recurring theme in this report, it's that buying the right shoe is an investment in foot health. But how do you find a shoe that fits properly and provides adequate support, without falling prey to commercial claims by shoe stores and manufacturers that may have no scientific basis?

Start with your own feet, and look at what's already in your closet. Stand barefoot on a piece of paper or cardboard, and trace the shape of each foot. Now take your shoes, one by one, and place them on top of the drawing. If you're like most people, your "comfortable" shoes will closely match the outline of your own feet. Identify the shoes that cause pain; most of these will be shoes with narrow toes or high heels, if you're a woman. Check to see if the toe of the shoe is narrower or shorter than your own foot.

Ideally, you would never wear shoes that are too small, too high, or too tight. But if you must have such shoes for special occasions, wear them as infrequently as possible or you'll increase your risk for foot pain and problems (or exacerbate those you already suffer). The less often you wear tight, ill-fitting shoes, the better. You might want to keep several pairs of shoes on hand; for instance, wearing comfortable, low-heeled pumps around the home or office or at casual gatherings, and saving high-heeled shoes for occasional dressy events.

Invest in good shoes

If you're able to afford it, consider investing in a few pairs of shoes that are good for your feet. Buying a pair that you can wear to work, another for dressy occasions, and a third for casual wear will put you in an ideal position to improve your foot health and do away with many pesky problems that are caused or exacerbated by pointy, tight shoes. Many manufacturers design shoes with both fashion and comfort in mind (see "Comfort analyzed," left). Some manufacturers promote special designs like air bubbles and composite materials (polyurethane, PVC, and the like) in soles to provide more cushioning.

There are a number of things you can look for when choosing a shoe (see "What to look for in a shoe," page 45). The bottom line is, how do you feel when you put them on? Trust what your feet tell you. You'll encounter a substantial amount of marketing hype from manufacturers; you can contact the American Podiatric Medical Association (APMA), or visit its website, to learn which manufacturers have been awarded the APMA Seal of Acceptance (see "Resources," page 47).

For women, the best shoes are low-heeled but not flat—no higher than three-quarters of an inch—with a wide padded heel, a wide toe box, and a sole that pro-

---

▶ **Comfort analyzed**

Shoe designs have exploded in creativity and style. Among the many fashionable choices, it is possible to find shoes that are both stylish and good for your feet. (For the names of shoe manufacturers that have earned the American Podiatric Medical Association's Seal of Acceptance, see "Resources," page 47, or visit the APMA website at www.apma.org.)

Men's shoes
Oxford-style shoes are among the best choices in footwear for men. (Oxfords also come in women's styles.) Look for a cushioned sole to provide support and a fit that's snug but not too tight. Heel pads, forefoot inserts, and other enhancements may also be added to further customize the fit.

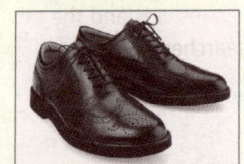

Image courtesy of The Rockport Company.

Women's shoes
Comfortable women's shoes can be attractive and stylish. Look for shoes with a low (but not flat), cushioned heel and a roomy toe box. Many shoes today are being designed with composition soles to offer extra shock absorption and enough room to accommodate custom orthoses.

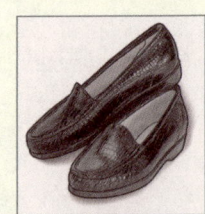

Image courtesy of SAS Shoes.

vides sufficient cushioning against the impact of walking. The height of a heel is more crucial than its width; in general, the higher the heel, the worse its effect on the foot. It doesn't matter whether the heel is thin and spiky or wide and chunky. One exception is when both toes and heel are raised high, as with platform shoes. Because both toes and heel are elevated, the toes are not subjected to additional stress. But watch your step in platform shoes: you may be more apt to twist your ankle.

Men generally feel most comfortable in athletic shoes, sturdy oxfords, wingtips, loafers, or low-heeled boots. Look for sturdy sole construction that provides support to the foot and cushions against shock. If you have weak or painful ankles, you may want to try a high-top sneaker or boot. If you have diabetes or rheumatoid arthritis, you may need special extra-depth shoes.

A few people benefit from shoes that are custom-designed to address a specific foot problem. People who have diabetes are more likely to fall into this category, as are those who have significant foot deformities. Discuss this option with your foot care specialist.

What to look for in a shoe

Both men and women benefit from shoes constructed from materials that breathe, which help keep the foot dry and less susceptible to foot fungus. The following steps may also be helpful:

1. Take a tracing of your foot with you when you go shopping. Place any shoe you think you might buy on top of the tracing. If it's narrower or shorter than the tracing, don't even try it on.

2. Wait until the afternoon to shop for shoes—your foot naturally expands with use during the day and may swell in hot weather.

3. Wear the same type of socks that you intend to wear with the shoes.

4. Have the salesperson measure both of your feet—and get measured every time you buy new shoes. Feet change with age, often growing larger and wider (as the accumulated weight they bear exacts its toll over time). If one foot is larger or wider than the other, buy a size that fits the larger foot.

FOOT FACTS for women

- About nine in 10 women wear shoes that are too small.
- About eight in 10 women wear shoes that are painful.
- Women are nine times more likely than men to develop a foot problem because of improperly fitting shoes.
- Tight shoes contribute to nine out of 10 foot problems in women.

Save flip-flops for the beach

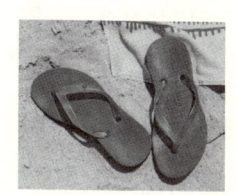

Planning to take a long walk? Need to get somewhere fast? You may want to leave your flip-flops in the dust, or at least choose a pair with the APMA seal of acceptance (see "Invest in good shoes," at left). Ordinary, flat-soled flip-flops pose some dangers to the foot. For example, scientists from Auburn University in Alabama who studied the biomechanics of flip-flops demonstrated that wearing flip-flops can actually cause foot pain and that they are not easy to walk in. What most people don't realize, and the research shows, is that they affect the way you walk—your walking gait—and that can lead to pain in the leg, right on up through the hip and lower back. What's more, flip-flop–related foot injuries, such as arch problems, sprained ankles, and tendinitis, are on the rise, according to the APMA.

The researchers evaluated 39 college-age men and women and divided them into two groups. One walked in flip-flops and the other wore athletic shoes. Researchers were able to measure vertical force of the feet, stride length, and leg angles. The people wearing flip-flops took shorter steps and walked with less vertical force than those wearing shoes. Those wearing flip-flops tended to grasp their toes and not raise their feet as much as the other group as they swung their legs forward, changes that affected ankle position and decreased stride length.

If you love wearing flip-flops in the summer, it's best to limit the amount of time you wear them. You could also invest in one of a number of athletic-styled flip-flops that offer sturdier construction and a contoured foot bed to support and fit your foot better than flat flip-flops—which aren't sturdy and offer no arch support. Look for flip-flops made of high-quality soft leather, which will minimize potential for blisters and other irritation, and make sure your foot doesn't hang off the edge of the shoe.

5. Stand in the shoes. Make sure you have at least a quarter- to a half-inch of space between your longest toe and the end of the shoe. This provides enough room for your foot to press forward as you walk, without jamming your toes. Wiggle your toes to make sure there's enough room, and press on the top of the shoe gently to determine where your longest toe lies.

6. Walk around in the shoes to determine how they feel. Is there enough room at the balls of the feet? Do the heels fit snugly, or do they pinch or slip off? Don't rationalize that the shoes just need to be "broken in" or that they'll stretch with time. Find shoes that fit from the start.

7. Trust your own comfort level rather than a shoe's size or description. Sizes vary from one manufacturer to another. And no matter how comfortable an advertisement claims those shoes are, you're the real judge.

8. Pay attention to width as well as length. If the ball of your foot feels compressed in a particular shoe, ask if it comes in a wider size. Buying shoes that are a half-size bigger—but no wider—won't necessarily solve the problem.

9. Feel the inside of the shoes to see if they have any tags, seams, or other material that might irritate your foot or cause blisters.

10. Turn the shoes over and examine the soles. Are they sturdy enough to provide protection from sharp objects? Do they provide any cushioning? Also, take the sole test as you walk around the shoe store: do the soles cushion against impact? Try to walk on hard surfaces as well as carpet to see how the shoe feels on both.

"Barefoot" running shoes

For decades, running shoes have been built with lots of cushioning and supporting structure. But now, some runners are looking for less shoe and more road feel. These "minimalist" runners maintain that running is a natural movement of the body and that the foot does not require heavy padding and bracing. Instead, they say these beefed-up shoes actually inhibit a runner's natural stride.

With this in mind, many running shoe companies now offer a minimalist model that promises a "closer-to-barefoot" running experience. These minimalist shoes are designed, in part, to shift the runner's landing position to the middle or front of the foot, thereby lessening the heavy impact of a heel landing.

Experts advise caution. Minimalist shoes may not be the right choice for everyone. The jury is still out on the benefits or adverse effects of these shoes. Your choice of shoe may depend on your natural gait. If you tend to land on your midfoot or forefoot, the minimalist shoes might be a good choice. If you naturally land on your heel, you may need the cushioning provided by a traditional running shoe. More research will be needed to answer a variety of questions, including whether less shoe equals more injuries, and also how these minimalist shoes affect performance.

Do you need orthoses?

Custom orthoses are designed to be placed in your shoe to correct or compensate for a structural problem that affects your foot, your gait, or both. But studies show that over-the-counter shoe inserts—the foam or silicone pads often sold in drugstores—are often just as effective and much less expensive. If you have foot discomfort in a particular pair of shoes, your first step should be to invest in better shoes (see "What to look for in a shoe," page 45). Properly fitted, well-cushioned shoes may provide you with the support you need. And since custom orthoses can vary widely in cost (ranging from $150 to $400), better-fitting shoes may be considerably less expensive. If you just need a little more cushioning, try an over-the-counter insert.

If the problem persists or if you find that you suffer discomfort in all of your shoes, talk to a foot care specialist.

Resources

Organizations

American Academy of Orthopaedic Surgeons
6300 N. River Road
Rosemont, IL 60018
800-346-2267 (toll-free)
www.aaos.org

This organization is primarily for doctors, but its website has extensive information written for lay people as well as a finder function for orthopedic surgeons.

American College of Foot and Ankle Surgeons
8725 W. Higgins Road, Suite 555
Chicago, IL 60631
800-421-2237 (toll-free)
www.footphysicians.com

This is the patient information site for the ACFAS, a professional organization of foot and ankle surgeons.

American Diabetes Association
1701 N. Beauregard St.
Alexandria, VA 22311
800-342-2383 (toll-free)
www.diabetes.org

This organization offers information on foot care for people with diabetes.

American Orthopaedic Foot and Ankle Society
6300 N. River Road, Suite 510
Rosemont, IL 60018
800-235-4855 (toll-free) or 847-698-4654 (outside United States)
www.aofas.org

This organization of foot and ankle specialists offers a foot care finder and extensive information on foot conditions on its website.

American Podiatric Medical Association
9312 Old Georgetown Road
Bethesda, MD 20814
800-275-2762 (toll-free)
www.apma.org

This organization for podiatrists offers an "Ask the Expert" function on its website to answer questions from the public about foot conditions and foot health.

Sock and shoe manufacturers

The American Podiatric Medical Association (see "Organizations," left) maintains an ongoing list of foot-healthy shoes, insoles, socks, and medications as part of its "Seal of Acceptance" and "Seal of Approval" programs. Listed below are some of the sock and shoe manufacturers on the APMA list (marked with asterisks), as well as other makers of comfortable, foot-friendly shoes and socks. For a complete list of the APMA-approved manufacturers, visit the organization's website at www.apma.org.

Aerosoles
201 Meadow Road
Edison, NJ 08817
800-798-9478 (toll-free)
www.aerosoles.com

Birkenstock
6 Hamilton Landing, Suite 250
Novato, CA 94948
800-867-2475 (toll-free)
www.birkenstock.com

*Dansko
8 Federal Road
West Grove, PA 19390
800-326-7564 (toll-free)
www.dansko.com

Easy Spirit
1129 Westchester Ave.
White Plains, NY 10604
888-327-9772 (toll-free)
www.easyspirit.com

*Ecco
16 Delta Drive
Londonderry, NH 03053
800-359-4399 (toll-free)
www.ecco.com

***Gold Toe Brands
(socks and hosiery)**
661 Plaid St.
Burlington, NC 27215
800-523-8265 (toll-free)
www.goldtoe.com

Mephisto Shoes
1026 North Blvd.
Oak Park, IL 60301
708-524-0321
www.mephistoshoes.com

Naturalizer Shoes
c/o Brown Shoe Company
8300 Maryland Ave.
St. Louis, MO 63105
888-294-1648 (toll-free)
www.naturalizeronline.com

*Rockport
700 Indian Springs Drive
Lancaster, PA 17601
866-290-6431 (toll-free)
www.rockport.com

SAS Shoemakers
1717 SAS Drive
San Antonio, TX 78224
877-782-7463 (toll-free)
www.sasshoes.com

Thor-Lo (athletic socks)
2210 Newton Drive
Statesville, NC 28677
888-846-7567 (toll-free)
www.thorlo.com

Glossary

Achilles' tendon: A band of connective tissue that runs up the back of the heel; susceptible to inflammation and rupture.

arthritis: Inflammation of a joint, often with destruction of cartilage. There are over 100 different types of arthritis.

athlete's foot: A fungal infection that causes a moist, itchy rash, usually between the toes or on the sole of the foot.

blister: A fluid-filled sac that develops between layers of skin, usually after prolonged irritation from an external source, like a shoe or the ground.

bunion: An angular deformity of the big toe, causing a bump to develop at its base; may become inflamed and painful.

bunionette: A condition similar to a bunion, but affecting the base of the fifth toe.

bursa: A fluid-filled sac that cushions a tendon near a bone.

bursitis: Inflammation of a bursa.

callus: An area of hardened skin that usually forms on the bottom of the feet to protect against irritation.

corn: An area of hardened skin that might have a dense knot in the center. Corns usually form on the toes because of irritation.

diabetes: A systemic condition in which a person's body is unable to convert sugars and other nutrients into energy. People with diabetes often experience foot disorders.

flat feet: A condition in which the arch is flat all the time (rigid flat feet) or flattens when bearing weight (flexible flat feet).

fracture: A broken bone.

fungus: A simple, plantlike organism that can infect such tissues as skin and nails; common fungal foot infections include athlete's foot and toenail fungus.

gait cycle: A description of the movement of your feet and legs while you walk, beginning when one heel strikes the ground and ending when that heel strikes the ground again a few seconds later.

gout: A type of arthritis that develops when uric acid, a normal byproduct of digestion, accumulates in the joints.

hammertoe: A sometimes painful condition in which the toe curls up and under (resembling a hammer).

heel spur: An abnormal growth of bone or calcium on the back or bottom of the heel bone.

ligament: Fibrous tissue that connects one bone to another.

melanoma: A kind of cancer that usually originates as a mole on the skin.

Morton's neuroma: A painful inflammation of a nerve in the foot that develops after compression, injury, or mechanical irritation.

neuropathy: Impaired nerve function due to systemic damage of the peripheral nerves; may result from diabetes.

orthopedist: A physician who specializes in musculoskeletal problems, including those of the bones, joints, tendons, and nerves.

orthoses: Custom shoe inserts, usually constructed of foam or a composite material; help cushion or realign the feet for people with foot deformities.

osteoarthritis: The most common type of arthritis; usually develops as a result of the wear and tear on joints over time.

plantar fascia: The ligament-like structure that connects the heel to the ball of the foot.

plantar fasciitis: An inflammation of the plantar fascia; the leading cause of heel pain.

podiatrist: A physician who specializes in the medical, surgical, and orthopedic management of foot and ankle disorders.

sesamoiditis: A painful inflammation in and around two small bones known as sesamoids, located under the head of the first metatarsal.

sprain: A tear in a ligament.

stress fracture: A hairline crack in a bone that usually occurs from overuse; left untreated, this may lead to displacement of the bones.

tendinitis: Inflammation of a tendon.

tendon: Sturdy tissue that connects a muscle to a bone.

vascular: Having to do with blood vessels and circulation.

wart: An abnormal fibrous growth caused by a viral infection.